GERIATRIC NURSING ASSISTANTS

GERIATRIC NURSING ASSISTANTS

An Annotated Bibliography with Models to Enhance Practice

George H. Weber

Bibliographies and Indexes in Gerontology, Number 12
Erdman B. Palmore, Series Adviser

Greenwood Press
New York • Westport, Connecticut • London

RC954
W3
1990

Library of Congress Cataloging-in-Publication Data

Weber, George H.
  Geriatric nursing assistants : an annotated bibliography with
models to enhance practice / George H. Weber.
      p. cm.—(Bibliographies and indexes in gerontology, ISSN
0743-7560 ; no. 12)
  Includes bibliographical references.
  Includes index.
  ISBN 0-313-26665-4 (lib. bdg. : alk. paper)
  1. Geriatric nursing. 2. Nurses' aides. 3. Geriatric nursing—
Bibliography. 4. Nurses' aides—Bibliography. I. Title.
II. Series.
  [DNLM: 1. Geriatric Nursing—methods—abstracts. 2. Nurses'
Aides—abstracts. ZWT 100 B5824 no. 12]
RC954.W3 1990
610.73'65—dc20
DNLM/DLC
for Library of Congress   90-3858

British Library Cataloguing in Publication Data is available.

Library of Congress Catalog Card Number: 90-3858
ISBN: 0-313-26665-4
ISSN: 0743-7560

First published in 1990

Greenwood Press, 88 Post Road West, Westport, CT 06881
An imprint of Greenwood Publishing Group, Inc.

Printed in the United States of America

The paper used in this book complies with the
Permanent Paper Standard issued by the National
Information Standards Organization (Z39.48-1984).

10 9 8 7 6 5 4 3 2 1

Dedicated to the nursing assistants who give so unselfishly of themselves to the elderly residents of nursing homes, many of whom are in such utter need.

Contents

Series Foreword

The annotated bibliographies in this series provide answers to the fundamental question, "What is known?" Their purpose is simple, yet profound: to provide comprehensive reviews and references for the work done in various fields of gerontology. They are based on the fact that it is no longer possible for anyone to comprehend the vast body of research and writing in even one subspecialty without years of work.

This fact has become true only in recent years. When I was an undergraduate (Class of '52) no one at Duke had even heard of gerontology. Almost no one in the world was identified as a gerontologist. Now there are over 6,000 professional members of the Gerontological Society of America. When I was an undergraduate there were no courses in gerontology. Now there are thousands of courses offered by most major (and many minor) colleges and universities. When I was an undergraduate there was only one gerontological journal (Journal of Gerontology, begun in 1945). Now there are over forty professional journals, and several dozen books on gerontology are published each year.

The reasons for this dramatic growth are well known: the large increase in numbers of aged, the shift from family to public responsibility for the security and care of the elderly, the recognition of aging as a "social problem," and the growth of science in general. It is less well known that this explosive growth in knowledge has created the need for new solutions to the old problem of comprehending and keeping up with a field of knowledge. The old indexes and library card catalogues have become increasingly inadequate for the job. On-line computer indexes and abstracts are one solution but do not make evaluative selections or organize sources logically as is done here. These annotated bibliographies are also more widely available than on-line computer indexes.

These bibliographies will obviously be useful for researchers who need to know what research has (or has not) been done in their field. The annotations contain enough information so that the researcher usually does not have to search out the original articles. In the past, the review of literature has often been haphazard and was rarely comprehensive, because of the large investment of time (and money) that would be required by a truly comprehensive review. Now, using these bibliographies, researchers can be more confident that they are not missing important previous research; they can be more confident that they are not duplicating past efforts and "reinventing the wheel." It may well become standard and expected practice for researchers to consult such bibliographies, even before they start their research.

These bibliographies will also be useful for academic geriatricians, practicing physicians, nurses, social workers, psychologists, physical therapists, pharmacists, nursing home administrators, and all other professionals working with older persons. Geriatrics is growing at a fast rate because of the great need for more health professionals adequately trained in geriatrics. This particular bibliography will be especially useful to nursing home administrators and others concerned with nursing homes because of its focus on geriatric nursing assistants.

Dr. Weber has done an outstanding job of covering all the relevant literature and organizing it into easily accessible form. Not only are there 223 annotated references organized into four chapters, but there are three chapters at the end about models to enhance the practice of geriatric nursing assistants.

There is also an author index and a comprehensive subject index with many cross-references for the items in the bibliography. Thus one can look for relevant material in this volume in several ways: (1) look up a given subject index; (2) look up a given author in the author index; or (3) turn to the chapter that covers the topic.

The annotations are written clearly and concisely so that the reader can quickly grasp the essence of the reference and easily decide whether to pursue it further or not.

So it is with great pleasure that we add this bibliography to our series. We believe you will find this volume to be the most useful, comprehensive, and easily accessible reference work in its field. I will appreciate any comments you care to send me.

Erdman B. Palmore
Center for the Study of Aging and Human Development
Box 3003, Duke University Medical Center
Durham, NC 27710

Acknowledgments

I wish to express gratitude to The National Catholic School of Social Services at The Catholic University of America for its interest in this project, particularly to the dean of the school, Dr. Frederick Ahearn, for making a sabbatical year possible. Some of that year was devoted to writing this publication. I also wish to express my appreciation to Dr. Betty Timberlake, who read and commented on an earlier version of this manuscript. Also, I wish to express gratitude to the many librarians in the Washington, D.C., area whom I consulted in the process of identifying the literature, particularly Mr. Larry Guthrie of the Nursing/Biology Library of The Catholic University. Also, my thanks go to two doctoral students in the School of Social Services-- Mr. Joseph Di Paolo and Mr. Gustavo Martinez--and a baccalaureate student--Ms. Roberta Gambale--for procuring many of the articles annotated in the document. Last, but certainly not least, I wish to acknowledge my appreciation to Dr. Erdman Palmore, Greenwood's gerontology series editor for his sage advice. Whatever oversights, errors, or shortcomings the book may have are those of the author.

Introduction

Increasing attention has been given to the nursing home care of the elderly in recent years (Institute of Medicine, 1986 and NCCNHR, 1988). This development has occurred under the stimulus of the growing number of old people in our society and society's tendency to overinstitutionalize people. Among the staff in nursing homes are the nursing assistants, who provide as much as 90 percent of the direct care provided the elderly. The nursing assistants are with the elderly around the clock doing a variety of tasks ranging from helping them to their toilet to comforting them during periods of distress.

The increasing interest has focused on nursing homes, but only on nursing assistants incidently as they are a part of the bigger nursing home picture. Their work is so important to the well-being of the residents that it suggested a book emphasizing the nursing assistants' psychosocial skills. Also, the scattered literature on nursing assistants including the literature pertinent to the construction of models to improve their practice needed pulling together and annotating.

The first four chapters present the annotated reviews. They are organized in anticipation of the construction of the models, which is the topic of Chapter 6. With this interest, the first four chapters review material on the tasks and context of the nursing assistants' work, and on ways to improve the nursing assistants' practice by training, organizational development, advocacy, and bargaining.

A psychosocial concept of nursing assistant practice is presented in Chapter 5, "Toward a Psychosocial Model of Practice." The caveat "toward" is used because the concept is tentative. It requires further development, especially detailing the various resident psychosocial circumstances (individual and group situations) to which the nursing assistant might respond helpfully and the various interventions or techniques that the nursing assistant might attempt. These responses and techniques must be tested for their helpfulness to the residents. Further, "toward" is used because administrators of nursing homes and directors of nursing must be convinced of the concept's utility in the nursing home's division of work, especially vis-à-vis tasks of the nurses.

Chapter 6 presents the intervention models--two on inservice training, two on organizational development, and one each on advocacy and bargaining. The models emphasize rigorous practice and its evaluation. They are presented in ideal-typical form but recognize the limitations of daily practice.

Chapter 7 discusses the activities necessary to develop the nursing assistant occupation, including political action. The moral aspects of moving ahead on an agenda for the nursing assistant are also considered.

The book aims to improve services to the nursing home residents. To do this, persons other than the nursing assistant--that is, administrators of nursing homes and directors of nursing--must address ways to improve the working conditions of nursing assistants, and academics must intensify their training, research, and advocacy efforts.

Last, the book hopes to encourage directors of training and direct supervisors of nursing assistants to help nursing assistants acquire the needed knowledge and skills.

I
The Nursing Assistant's Job

An annotated bibliography of published works about nursing assistants in nursing homes for the elderly follows in this and the next three chapters. Some related pertinent literature is also annotated. For example, some material on psychiatric nursing assistants is included in the nursing assistant's job literature. Several references on educational theory are included in Chapter 3. A number of books on general advocacy and bargaining are in the advocacy and bargaining material. Also, several articles on research instruments are included in Chapters 1 and 2 because of their potential to evaluate training and other models.

The items--articles, books, and dissertations--included in the bibliography were generated from the following sources: Cumulative Index to Nursing and Allied Health Literature (volumes 1980-1988); Current Literature on Aging (volumes 1980-1989), published by the National Council on the Aging; bibliographies in the Institute of Medicine's Improving the Quality of Care in Nursing Homes (1986), and in the National Citizens' Coalition for Nursing Home Reform's Final Report, Nurse Aide Training Symposium (1988), and Dissertation Abstracts International (years 1971-1986). Also, the Medline retrieval source generated a number of references.

The search of bibliographic resources included The Catholic University of America's Nursing/Biology Library, the National Library of Medicine, the U.S. Public Health Parklawn Health Services Library, the National Gerontology Resource Center of the American Association of Retired Persons, the National Council on Aging Library, and the Service Employee International Union--AFL-CIO. Though less formal, the process of reviewing the material identified by the aforementioned sources lead to additional references. That process generated a richer and wider literature than was initially expected. Further, the review was initially intended to cover approximately ten years--1980 to the present; however, it turned out to cover a much longer period. The earliest article reviewed dates back to 1953.

The nursing assistant's job is directly linked to the residents and their welfare. Though knowledge and skill are required to perform its tasks, the nursing assistant's job is often viewed as one that can be performed by the exercise of everyday skills and humanitarian attitudes. Yet it is a complex one, requiring technical knowledge and skill as well as diligence, hard work, and commitment to the personal care of residents.

BOOKS

1. National Institute of Mental Health (1965). The psychiatric aide in state mental hospitals. Washington, D.C.: U.S. Government Printing Office. 113 Pp.

    This report covers a number of basic areas on psychiatric aides, including: their number and demographic characteristics, salary and working conditions, job duties and job attitudes, training facilities and practices, and nurses' attitudes toward aides.

2. Quinlin, A. (1988). Chronic care workers: Crisis among paid caregivers of the elderly. Washington, D.C.: Older Women's League and AFSCME, AFL-CIO. 31 Pp.

    This monograph records the crisis among paid caregivers of the elderly, most of whom work in nursing homes. The job turnover is very high. Among the reasons are: low pay, poor benefits, inadequate training, stressful working conditions, few opportunities to advance, and low status in the health care hierarchy. Statistical projections show 500,000 new nursing aides and home health care workers will be employed by the year 2000. However, wages for these workers are not likely to increase rapidly. The major policy question that faces long-term care providers is how to staff long-term care facilities with well-trained caregivers with equitable compensation.

JOURNALS

3. Ashton, V., and Barrett, V. (1983). "Effective strategies to control disturbing behavior." Nursing Homes, 32(4):18-21.

   Eighteen general guidelines are provided to cope with residents' disturbing behaviors such as repetitious speech, stealing, withdrawal, resistance, lack of cleanliness, wandering, demanding behavior, delusions, refusal to eat, refusal to follow medical orders, suicidal tendencies, and physically or verbally assaultive behavior.

4. Balz, T. M., and Turner, J. G. (1977). "Development and analysis of nursing home aide screening device." The Gerontologist, 17(1):66-69.

   This article reports the development, testing, and analysis of a nursing home aide screening device. Following its development, the instrument was administered to a sample of employed aides who were rated by supervisors as successful or unsuccessful. Forty items of the instrument were found to differentiate significantly between the two groups of aides. Further testing with larger samples is necessary.

5. Beach, D. A. (1988). "Health care providers inventory; a method for evaluating nursing aides." Journal of Psychology, 122(1):89-94.

   Beach, D. A. (1988). "A new procedure in the evaluation of nursing aide applicants." Nursing Homes and Senior Citizen Care, 37(2):17-18.

   These two articles describe the Health Care Provider Inventory (HCPI), a preemployment instrument. It is a seventy-item questionnaire with five major scales that measure: ability to relate to nursing home residents, ability to communicate clearly and courteously, willingness to assist other staff, appropriate attitudes to provide services in a health care setting, and prospective adequacy to work as an employee in a nursing home. It can be administered in twenty minutes. Limited research suggests promise; however, more study is needed.

6. Bier, R. I. (1961). "Rehabilitation on a shoestring." American Journal of Nursing, 61(8):98-100.

Inspiration, initiative, planning, and perseverance by the nursing supervisor and the nursing home's physician in charge of physical medicine and rehabilitation staff were instrumental in the initiation and conduct of a rehabilitation program. Staff, including nursing assistants, had their jobs refined to focus on rehabilitative functions. Further, they were motivated to deliver their best skills, and were recognized for their contribution.

7. Brannon, D., et al. (1988). "A job diagnostic survey of nursing home caregivers: Implications for job redesign." The Gerontologist, 28(2):246-252.

Nursing home caregiving was analyzed as a job. Information from interviews with administrators was combined with survey data from 489 nursing assistants and LPNs in twenty-one nursing homes. The study sought information to assess the need for, and feasibility of, redesigning caregiving work. Implementation principles and examples were included.

8. Brown, M. (1988). "Nursing assistants' behavior toward the institutionalized elderly." Quarterly Review Bulletin (QRB), 14(1):15-17.

Twenty-seven randomly selected nursing assistants were drawn from a long-term care facility to determine the relationship between their behavior toward residents and their opinions about inservice training programs, their perceptions of their supervisors, and their attitudes toward the elderly. Separate questionnaires were used to generate information from the nursing assistants and their supervisors. Regression analysis indicated a positive relationship between the nursing assistants' behavior toward the residents and the nursing assistants' opinions about inservice training, perceptions of their supervisors, and attitudes to the elderly. Suggestions for further study of these matters were made.

9. Bye, M. G., and Iannone, J. (1987). "Excellent care-givers of the elderly: What satisfies them about their work." Nursing Homes, 36(4):36-39.

The aim of this study was to identify the items that satisfy excellent nursing assistants, and to determine whether their reasons for beginning work with the sick elderly were the same as those for remaining on the job. The sample consisted of thirty nursing assistants selected by the directors of nursing from three types of nursing homes: private, proprietary, and church-affiliated. The homes' turnover rates were mixed, as were their types of residents. The criteria of caregiver excellence were: consistently giving safe, efficient, and effective care to patients; and displaying a caring attitude in patient-care encounters. The subjects were asked in a guided interview to list their tasks from the most to the least desirable. They were also asked: (1) What attracted you to this type of work when you first began? and (2) Are the reasons you started to work in long-term care the same reasons that are keeping you here? Eight questions were asked to get demographic information on the nursing assistants. Content analysis was used to analyze the information. The reasons given for beginning to work with the sick elderly included: (1) having had very positive role models, (2) deeply felt need to help other people, particularly older people, (3) always wanted to be a nurse and the job was a steppingstone to becoming a nurse, or allowing me to do nurselike work, and (4) needed a job and it was the first job I could find. Of the nursing assistants who started working in long-term care because of a love of older people, or of a love of nursing, or because of positive role models, all reported staying in long-term care for the same reasons. They felt committed to the work, and enjoyed working with elderly people. These were somewhat different from the initial reasons for seeking the job.

10. Dawes, P. L. (1981). "The nurses' aide and the team approach in the nursing home." Journal of Geriatric Psychiatry, 14(2):265-276.

This is a candid essay that examines whether nursing assistants' participation in team meetings that typically include administrators, physicians, nurses, and adjunctive therapists would improve the nursing assistants' jobs and working conditions. Suggested positive gains included improved relations to other staff, patient care, and self-esteem. However, these were seen as marginal because they are unlikely to offset the nursing assistants' basic problems: (1) inadequate staffing, (2) the nursing home's deep-seated prejudice that puts the nursing assistant at the bottom of the home's professional-nonprofessional hierarchy, (3) the nursing assistant's lack of verbal and paramedical skills, and (4) unreasonably and unjustly low material compensation.

11. Erickson, J. (1987). "Quality and the nursing assistant." Provider, 13(4):4-6.

Skilled selection, orientation, and training of nursing assistants and recognizing their good work are viewed as prudent nursing home management procedures in this article.

12. Fisk, V. R. (1984). "When nurses' aides care." Journal of Gerontological Nursing, 10(3):121-127.

This is a study that sought to answer: (1) how nursing assistants view themselves as part of a nursing home organization, (2) how nursing assistants view the elderly people for whom they care, and (3) how nursing assistants view the care they give residents. These broad questions were pursued by detailed questions about: personal qualities needed to work as a nursing assistant; reasons for the transfer of nursing assistants to non-nursing care jobs; and the proper care for incontinent residents, and for noisy residents. A convenience sample of thirty nursing assistants was taken from a 165-bed philanthropic home (twenty subjects) and a 34-bed proprietary home (ten subjects). The data included demographic information and responses to a twenty-four-item open-ended interview on the above questions. The study's findings were: patience and understanding were required of nursing assistants; and job changes occurred because working with nursing home residents, particularly confused and incontinent residents. The findings also indicated that intrastaff conflicts were disruptive, and the complaints of residents' families were anxiety arousing. The implications of the study included: training of nursing assistants; their increased responsibility for resident care; and encouragement of the nursing assistants' sense of personal worth and self-image.

13. Floyd, G. J. (1983). "A job satisfaction profile: Psychiatric nursing aides." Nursing Management, 14(9):36-40.

Two hundred thirteen nursing aides from one state hospital answered a questionnaire to determine the factors that influenced their work satisfactions. The factors identified were ability to help others, complete recovery of patients, presence of good medical staff, opportunity to move up to a better position, adequate equipment, sufficient personnel, and periodic increases in salary.

14. Friedman, S. (1975). "A resident welcoming committee: Institutionalized elderly in volunteer services to their peers." The Gerontologist, 15(5):362-367.

This is a descriptive report of a resident welcoming committee, established and assisted by a facility social worker. Composed initially of twelve alert residents, the group worked diligently, making several visits a week to new residents. An evaluation after twelve weeks suggested the committee was achieving its objectives: providing peer support for newly admitted residents; affording opportunities for longer-term residents to perform volunteer work; and creating a forum for the volunteers to discuss their work.

15. Gale, C. B. (1973). "Walking in the aide's shoes." American Journal of Nursing, 73(4):628-631.

This research reports the account of a trained nurse who worked as a nursing assistant (participant observer) for four months. Impressions of the aides' feelings about their jobs, working conditions, and lack of regard by the nurses and administrators are presented, as well as the author's personal reactions as a participant observer.

16. Giviel, L., Linn, M. W., and Linn, B. S. (1972). "Physical and mental impairment-of-function evaluation in the aged: The PAMIE Scale." Journal of Gerontology, 27(1):83-90.

This article reports the development and use of the PAMIE as an instrument for the quantitative description of a wide range of behaviors pertinent to the adult chronically ill generally and to the institutionalized geriatric patient specifically. The rationale and statistical data on the scale's development are presented.

17. Handschu, S. S. (1973). "Profile of the nurse's aide: Expanding her role as psycho-social companion to the nursing home resident." The Gerontologist, 31(17):315-317.

Interviews with 206 nurse's aides chosen at random from the day and afternoon shifts at forty nursing homes in the greater Detroit area showed that most were paid less than $80.00 per week at the time of the study, and that only two-thirds of them were given any on-the-job training. The sample was stratified and weighted to represent the actual proportion of beds by size of home, type of home ownership, and percentage of residents with public support. Each aide was interviewed for about forty-five minutes by a field worker who had spent two or three days observing in the nursing home. Findings included: 49 percent of the aides were high school graduates and, of those, 81 percent were under twenty five years of age; slightly more than half of the aides had taken academic courses outside their current jobs; and only about a dozen of these 106 aides took geriatric or gerontology courses. Many of the nursing homes had inservice training, but the training was limited to refresher courses in basic nursing care.

18. Hawthorn, P. J. (1987). "An aide or a hindrance." Nursing Times, 83(1):56.

Project 2000, a British initiative to upgrade health care services, specified that the job of an aide/auxiliary should be developed to assist in the care of patients. This article is critical of the concept because of its lack of clarity about what the auxiliary is to do, and how her duties would fit in with the current structure of services. Further, the article raises the question of who is to train this category of workers so they are competent to perform whatever duties they are assigned.

19. Henderson, J. N. (1987). "When a professor turns nurse aide." Provider, 13(4):8-12.

This is a brief but insightful report by an academic who spent thirteen months as a nursing assistant in a ninety-bed proprietary nursing home. The staff and residents were aware of his identity. The fact that he was actually performing the work of a nursing assistant did not distort the behavior of either staff or residents, in his view. The experience gave him great empathy and respect for the contribution of the nursing assistant, especially because of her inadequate pay and heavy work load.

20. Holder, E. L. (1987). "The nursing assistant: To know quality is to give it." Provider, 13(4):36-37.

This article gives emphasis to the contribution of nursing assistants to quality care. The exceptional demands on the nursing assistants are pointed out and factors to retain them on the job such as basic training and continuing education are noted. A standard national training program for nursing assistants is urged. That suggestion asks the Social Security Act to be amended requiring all states to train and test nursing assistants.

21. Holz, G. A. (1982). "Nursing aides in nursing homes: Why are they satisfied?" Journal of Gerontological Nursing, 8(5):265-271.

Using a convenience sample drawn mostly from one facility, this study tapped thirty-one subjects for their views on ten factors and their relationship to staying with their job. The factors were: peer and supervisory relationships, achievement, the work itself, responsibility, salary, recognition, administrative policies, working conditions, and advancement. Results indicated that interpersonal relationships were the most important. Next in importance were achievement, and responsibility. Work itself was reported the fifth of the ten factors. Salary, recognition, administrative policies, working conditions, and advancement followed. A recommendation was made for a more representative study.

22. Howard, E. (1974). "The effect of work experience in a nursing home on the attitudes toward death held by nurse aides." The Gerontologist, 14(1):54-56.

Even though nursing assistants must constantly deal with the problems of death and dying, this small study of twenty-eight white nursing assistants chosen because of their availability from seven nursing homes in an unspecified location indicated their avoidance of death and dying issues. An interview schedule composed of thirteen basic questions was used. Several illustrative questions follow: (1) Would you be willing to discuss your feelings about death with a patient, if he were to ask? (2) How do you feel about conversations about death between patients? (3) Do you feel that most patients fear death, avoid all thoughts of death, or long for death? Attitudinal training was suggested as a means to encourage nursing assistants to recognize death as a nursing home reality.

23. Jones, P. L., and Millman, A. (1986). "A three-part system to combat pressure sores." Geriatric Nursing, 7(2):78-82.

This article encourages assessing the nature, extent, and probable causal factors of pressure sores, and developing an individual plan of care for each resident. Careful implementation and followup of the plan are also suggested. Possibilities for research are provided.

24. Kahl, A. (1976). "Special jobs for special needs: An overview."
    Occupational Outlook Quarterly, 20(3):2-5.

    A greater number of workers will be required, into the next
    century, to meet the various psychological, social, financial, and
    medical needs of an increasing number of elderly people in the
    American society. Rapid increases are occurring in both the
    number and proportion of persons over seventy-five. This elderly
    subgroup needs much more assistance, on the whole, than those
    who are younger. By the year 2000, 13.5 million Americans will
    be over seventy-five. Nursing homes will be challenged to meet
    the needs of people requiring their care.

25. Klus, G. W., and Thoreson, E. H. (1980). "The nurses aide: A
    life of uncertainty." Nursing Homes, 29(2):2-8.

    This is a qualitative descriptive report on stress experienced by
    nursing assistants. Twenty-five nursing assistants were selected
    randomly from two nursing homes. The responses were laden
    with feelings and indicated that their nursing home life was
    saturated with grievances, absenteeism, turnover, and employee
    distress. Five major sources of conflict were identified between:
    residents and their families, nursing assistants and their peers,
    nursing assistants and personnel in other departments, nursing
    assistants and their supervisors, and nursing assistants and the
    requirements of the job. Strategies to make appropriate changes
    were encouraged.

26. Ledet, J., Dangerfield, E., and Robinson, M. (1987). "Speaking
    from the 'Cajun Country' South." Provider, 13(4):28-30.

    The reflections of three nursing assistants indicated their major
    job frustrations stemmed from the lack of time to spend with
    individual residents, insufficient number of nursing assistants to
    do the required work, and that even the best of care may not
    result in the residents' improvement. They suggest improved
    recruiting procedures aimed at hiring mature, sensitive, and caring
    people, and an increased number of nursing assistant job slots to
    improve the situation.

27. LeSar, K. W. (1987). "Who provides for the nursing assistant?"
    Provider, 13(4):20-22.

Administrators, licensed nurses, long-term care organizations, and nursing assistants are urged to work toward recognizing and promoting the position of nursing assistant as a creditable and rewarding career. Intensified recruitment, improved working conditions, uniform training procedures, career ladders, and increased regard for nursing assistants are suggested as ways to improve the care of nursing home residents.

28. McKinley, M., Bodnar, P., and Swift, L. (1987). "Speaking from the heart of the midwest." Provider, 13(4):24-26.

Written by three nursing assistants, this article cites the satisfactions and frustrations of the job. Recommendations are made to administrators, specifically: reduce the case load of residents assigned to the nursing assistant; provide a career ladder of employment and a retirement pension plan; develop a method of preventing job burnout; create a training program for nursing assistants with the active involvement of nursing assistants; create a teaching position for a nursing assistant, and demonstrate a greater regard for nursing assistants.

29. Michocki, R. J., and Lamy, P. P. (1976). "The care of decubitus ulcers (pressure sores)." Journal of the American Geriatrics Society, 24(5):217-224.

Pressure sores remain a difficult problem in nursing homes. Management of these sores requires cleanliness, dryness, relief of pressure, and exposure to air. Other therapies that may be used are: proteolytic enzymes, surgical debridement, gold leaf, and various ointments.

30. Mueller, D. J., and Atlas, L. (1972). "Resocialization of regressed elderly residents: A behavioral management approach." Journal of Gerontology, 27(3):390-392.

Five male subjects ranging in age from fifty to eighty-two years were selected on the basis of their being ambulatory, in reasonable touch with reality, capable of conversation (although generally isolated), willing to attend group sessions, and relatively free of heavy sedation to participate in a behavioral management procedure. The goal was to "guide" the subjects back to some semblance of appropriate social give-and-take behavior from a withdrawn isolated state. The procedures included eleven group sessions in which interaction was encouraged and reinforced. Refreshments were also provided. Each session lasted thirty to thirty-five minutes. The interaction of the subjects increased appreciatively during the eleven sessions. Staff reported a carryover of increased conversation on the living units.

31. Myrtle, R. C. (1982). "Are nurse aides satisfied with their supervisors?" American Health Care Association Journal, 8(6):17-21.

Eighty-three workers representing slightly more than 25 percent of the nonsupervisory, nonprofessional staff of four long-term care institutions were selected at random. They completed a 197-item questionnaire to determine the conditions that influence a worker's feeling of satisfaction with her supervisor. The research findings suggested that the climate of the organization and the responses of the supervisor to the needs of the workers were the major determinants of the worker's satisfaction with their supervisors.

32. Nacapuy, C., Aezon, M., and Labrador, M. (1987). "Speaking from the Island Oahu." Provider, 13(4):26-28.

Written by three nursing assistants, this article speaks of the personal satisfactions of helping others; recommends reducing the nursing assistants' case load of residents to allow the nursing assistants more time to attend to the personal care of the residents; suggests improving the salary and fringe benefits of the nursing assistants to match their responsibilities; and proposes involving nursing assistants in the recruitment of other nursing assistants.

33. Parry, B. T. (1971). "Nurses' aides." Nursing Homes, 20(5):36-37.

The nursing assistants' intuitive knowledge and skill are recognized and nursing homes are urged to give them greater pay and involvement in the decision making regarding resident care.

34. Rinke, C. L., Williams, J. J., Lloyd, K. E., and Smith-Scott, W. (1978). "The effects prompting and reinforcement on self-bathing by elderly residents of a nursing home." Behavior Therapy, 9(5):873-881.

Prompting and reinforcement, first in combination and then separated, were applied to the self-bathing of four elderly nursing home residents while two other residents served as untreated controls. The steps of bathing were divided into five units: undressing, soaping, rinsing, drying, and dressing. Results indicated the experimental procedures (prompting and reinforcement) led to improved bathing behavior.

35. Sand, P., and Berni, R. (1974). "An incentive contract for nursing home aides." American Journal of Nursing, 74(3):475-477.

The base rates of residents' activities (positioning in bed, sitting on a chair or on a wheelchair, walking, conversing, and participating in recreational activities) in a living unit were computed by a research observer. A second observer demonstrated a high reliability of the base rates. Eight residents were randomly selected from this living unit as the experimental group and the eight remaining residents served as the control group. Incentive contracts were presented and accepted by the nursing assistants working with the experimental group of residents. The arrangement with the nursing assistants working with the control group was not clear. Three weeks of intervention followed with the experimental group. The nursing assistants encouraged the experimental group to increase their activities. Also, project staff had one fifteen-minute instructional meeting with the nursing assistants during each treatment week. Further, the occupational and speech therapists and nursing supervisors served as consultants to the nursing assistants. Bonuses were distributed weekly to the nursing assistants and residents as per the contracts. Of the eight persons in the experimental groups, five showed statistically significant improvement in activities. The patients not on the incentive program also appeared to show small changes toward more activity. A two-week followup showed a continuation of these achievements.

36. Sandel, S. L., and Johnson, D. R. (1987). "Nursing staff attitudes toward the work environment in a skilled nursing facility." Nursing Homes and Senior Citizen Care, 36(4):16-20.

This article reports the attitudes of nursing staff toward their work environments in one long-term facility. Management strategies are suggested to improve morale and job performance.

37. Schnelle, J. F., and Traughber, B. (1983). "A behavioral assessment
     system applicable to geriatric nursing facility residents." Behavioral
     Assessment, 5(3):231-243.

     Nursing assistants rated residents' behaviors on a monthly basis.
     Through computer assistance, nursing assistants' ratings were
     organized to identify potential goals for rehabilitation programs,
     track changes in resident behaviors over time, and identify
     institutionwide patterns of behavioral functioning and behavioral
     change. This system was evaluated by having nursing assistants rate
     behaviors of more than 200 residents in three different facilities
     over a full year. High interrater reliability was maintained over
     this period. Validity of the nursing assistants' ratings was high.
     They were correlated to the residents' behavior as observed by
     independent observers. The instrument used by the researchers--
     The Geriatric Assessment Inventory--tapped seven areas: self-help
     (general), self-help (eating), depression, socialization,
     communication, locomotion, and cognitive/memory functioning.

38. Sheridan, J. E., Fairchild, T. J., and Kaas, M. (1983). "Assessing
     the job performance of nursing home staff." Nursing Research,
     32(2):102-107.

     This article describes the development of the Behavioral Anchored
     Rating Scales (BARS) to measure the job performance of
     individual nurses and nursing assistants. The job performance
     dimensions for nursing assistants were: job knowledge and
     judgment, observational skills, job dependability, cooperation, and
     interpersonal skills. The scales reliability was tested to be very
     high.

39. Slack, P. (1986). "Project 2000: Whose helping hand?" Nursing
     Times, 82(29):33-34.

     Auxiliaries (nursing assistants) have been working in British
     hospitals for thirty years and in the community for ten. Project
     2000 accepts the need for such staff but rejects the idea that they
     should be in large numbers. Many nurses fear that nursing
     assistants will fill vacancies left by enrolled (registered) nurses and
     care will be attempted by untrained auxiliaries. This essay reviews
     the proposed training for the nursing assistants and suggests the
     nursing profession may have to consider working with nursing

assistants as part of the health care team because of the contributions that nursing assistants can make.

40. Spangler, P. F., Risley, T. R., and Belyew, D. D. (1984). "The management of dehydration and incontinence in nonambulatory geriatric patients." Journal of Applied Behavior Analysis, 17(3):397-401.

The nursing care procedures for nonambulatory dehydrated and incontinent residents were analyzed and new procedures were developed including highly specific instructions and recording techniques for nursing assistants. The new procedures had positive results on continence and hydration levels. Moreover, the researchers demonstrated that their approach could be incorporated into existing nursing care procedures.

41. Stricklan, P., Einhorn, V., and Jones, C. (1987). "Characteristics of nursing staff in long-term-care facilities: Their training, experience, and perceived proficiency levels." Nursing Homes, 36(1):22-27.

Aiming to establish a profile of nursing employees (124 aides, seventeen LPNs, and ten RNs drawn from six skilled nursing homes for a total of 158 nursing personnel), this study used the Employee Profile Sheet and Facility Profile Sheet. The major elements of the study were eleven selected practice areas and the several categories of nursing personnel responses to them. The nursing assistants (along with the LPNs) saw themselves as most qualified to attend to the overall well-being of residents, but they did not see themselves as qualified to care for the terminally ill or the mentally ill.

42. Wagnild, G., and Manning, R. W. (1985). "Convey respect during bathing procedures." Journal of Gerontological Nursing, 11(12):6-10.

This project sought to demonstrate the effectiveness of quasi-experimental bathing procedures involving forty-two residents in eight geriatric long-term care facilities. Though more detailed information and further study are needed, the importance of respect for the residents in helping them bathe is affirmed.

43. Wagnild, G., and Manning, R. W. (1986). "Screening and selecting applicants for nurse's aide." The Journal of Long-Term Care Administration, 14(2):2-4.

This study generated from interview data on 119 nursing assistants (all females) and approximately 47 percent of all full-time nursing assistants in a central Texas facility suggests that high-turnover persons (those who leave within a year) are less than twenty-eight of age, not married, and trained or educated beyond the job's requirements. Also their employment histories indicate that they are more likely to have had less than eighteen months in previous positions, and worked in two or more nursing homes within a three year period.

DISSERTATION

44. Harrington, V. L. (1982). "Nursing assistants on the night shift in a nursing home: Motivations and adaptations." M.A. Thesis, Department of Anthropology, The Catholic University of America, Washington, D.C., 98 Pp.

This research, conducted by a registered nurse working as an anthropological field researcher (she combined part-time nightshift work as a nurse in a nonprofit nursing home with being a scientific observer), provides a vivid description of the shared culture of nursing assistants on the night shift. Cultural theory, role theory, and systems theory were used to analyze the complex problems encountered by the nursing assistants. In addition to this analysis, the author also considered the stress of the job and its working conditions, particularly its poor pay and lack of respect.

SUMMARY

Because of the physical, functional, and mental disabilities of the residents, the job of the nursing assistant is demanding. Moreover, the nursing assistant's lack of training, heavy work load, and general low regard make the job increasingly difficult. The psychosocial aspect of the job is given some attention; however, it is not developed.

II
The Work Environment of the Nursing Assistant and Its Development

The formal and informal administrative components of the nursing home organization, the physical aspects of the place, and the composition of the staff and residents make up the work environment of nursing assistants.

Organizational development concerns upgrading the nursing home's structure to enhance the residents' care, and improve the job of nursing assistants. Such development may include a range of things, including improved decision making about the care of the residents, improved communication to and from management, improved visiting arrangements for friends and relatives of the residents, improved career opportunities for nursing assistants, and research on the quality of service.

BOOKS

45. Bennett, C. (1980). <u>Nursing home life: What it is and what it could be</u>. New York: Tiresias Press. 192 Pp.

This book has a unique perspective, having been written by one who has been both a nursing home administrator and a resident -- the latter as a participant observer who stayed ten days as a resident and whose identity was kept secret from all but the top-level staff. Yet the book is neither an anecdotal report of his first-hand experiences nor a sociological field report about a unique subculture. Rather, it is a report on the quality of care offered by several nursing homes and makes recommendations to improve them.

46. Brager, G., and Holloway, S. (1978). Changing human service organizations: Politics and practice. New York: The Free Press. 244 Pp.

Using Kurt Lewin's field theory and aspects of organizational theory, this book develops a strategy for employees at the rank-and-file level, and without any formal authority or responsibility to initiate change. The strategy suggests a Lewinian "force-field" analysis of the situation targeted for change as a way of understanding the forces that would support and those that would resist change. Techniques for gaining support include persuasion, participating on agency committees, conferring with others, and appealing to professional ethics and values. These techniques are viewed as belonging to one of the following categories of tactics: collaboration, campaign, and contest. Recognition is given to possible disapproval by the organization's administration, uncertain legitimacy, fear of reprisal, and threat to job security.

47. Burger, S., Miller, B., and Mauney, B. F. (1986). A guide to management and supervision of nursing homes. Springfield, Ill.: Charles C. Thomas. 531 Pp.

Though written for persons responsible for establishing a new nursing home, this comprehensive text should also be of help to those administering ones already in operation. The topics of the twenty-seven chapters range from administration and financial management to organization of resident activity.

48. Dailey-Murray, M. (1988). The new long term care survey process: A facility guide. Owings Mills, Md.: National Health Publishing. 185 Pp.

This handbook is based on the regulations for Medicare and Medicaid facility surveys published by the Department of Health and Human Services, Health Care Finance Administration. Organized as a "cookbook," it lists all of the elements necessary to meet the regulations. The following areas are covered: nursing, dietary, social services, resident activities, physical environment, resident rights, pharmacy, specialized rehabilitation services, laboratory and radiologic services, infection control, and medical records. A history of the survey process in long-term care facilities and how the new process came into being are described. Appendices include a number of forms to conduct a survey.

49. Donabedian, A. (1980). <u>The definitions of quality and approaches to its assessment</u>. Ann Arbor, Mich.: Health Administration Press. 163 Pp.

This book deals with the quality of medical care and its assessment. The material is presented in three parts. The first part is a conceptual exploration of the definition of quality. It considers quantity of care and its quality, monetary cost, benefits, accessibility, and practitioner satisfaction. The second part is concerned with empirical studies, particularly studies on the clients' view of quality, the providers' view of quality, and comparisons of the views of clients and providers. Part three focuses on the approaches to assessment and considers evaluating the process and outcome of medical care. Also, matters of ethics, values, and social policy are discussed.

50. Fivars, G., and Gosnell, D. (1966). <u>Nursing evaluation: The problem and the process</u>. Pittsburgh, Penn.: Westinghouse Learning Corporation. 228 Pp.

The book describes the application of the critical incident approach for evaluating nursing home care. Considerable attention is given to establishing broad, overall institutional objectives, developing curricula consistent with the institutional objectives, and selecting learning experiences designed to meet the students' educational needs. These considerations are organized by the step-by-step procedures of the critical incident approach and culminate in a presentation of the use of that approach in evaluating the performance of nursing care.

51. French, W. L., and Bell, C. H., Jr. (1984). <u>Organization development: Behavioral science interventions for organization improvement</u>. Third edition. Englewood Cliffs, N.J.: Prentice-Hall. 347 Pp.

This is a highly developed work in organization development that covers a broad range of topics, for example, key issues in the field, theory, and practices in a variety of settings, and future trends.

52. George, L. K. (editor) (1980). Quality of care in nursing homes:
     Attitudinal and environmental factors.   Durham, N.C.:   Duke
     University Press. 270 Pp.

     This volume reports the design and results of a study conducted
     to examine the organizational and personal factors that contribute
     to job turnover, job satisfaction, intentions to remain in the current
     job, and absenteeism among staff members at long-term care
     institutions.   The conceptual model used posited that these
     employment-related outcomes would be influenced by four sets of
     independent variables: (1) characteristics of the work place (size,
     staffing patterns), (2) specific job characteristics (pay, fringe
     benefits) and personal factors (age, marital status) of staff
     members, (3) perceptions of the social climate of the work
     environment, and (4) relevant social psychological attitudes
     (attitudes toward aging). The data base consisted of organizational
     data from fifteen long-term care institutions and surveys from 469
     staff members of these facilities. Surveys were administered to the
     three types of nursing personnel with the greatest responsibility for
     direct patient care: (1) registered nurses, (2) licensed practical
     nurses, and (3) nurses aides, orderlies, and other patient care
     assistants. As expected, annual turnover rates in this sample were
     high, ranging from a low of 55.3 percent for full-time registered
     nurses to a high of 145.1 percent among part-time nurses aides.

53. Glasscote, R., et al. (1976). Old folks at homes. Washington,
     D.C.: American Psychiatric Association. 148 Pp.

     The material for this report was generated by survey procedures,
     review of documents, and visits by teams of psychiatric experts to
     ninety-one facilities including skilled, intermediate, and mixed
     nursing homes, and bed and board care homes. The objective was
     to determine the quality of care provided the elderly, including the
     mentally ill elderly, in these settings. Chapters on these topics,
     vignettes of programs, and recommendations to improve the care
     of elderly are presented.

54. Granger, C. V., and Gresham, G. E. (editors) (1984). Functional
     assessment in rehabilitation medicine. Baltimore, Md.: Williams
     & Wilkins. 407 Pp.

     This edited volume contains twenty-two chapters authored or
     coauthored by experts in their topical areas. Its focus is on the

functional assessment of disabled persons and on the application of the assessment procedure to the rehabilitation of the disabled. The scope of the book is substantial, and its detail is comprehensive as its chapters cover a range of topics including the conceptualization and operationalization of functional assessment and the debilitating conditions to which such assessment is applicable; issues involved in measuring disability; instruments for documenting outcomes in rehabilitation; and research applications of functional assessment instruments in rehabilitation medicine. Two chapters focus on the elderly: one is on the functional assessment of aged persons and the other is on assessing the formal and informal support systems in high-risk elderly populations.

55. Gubrium, J. F. (1975). Living and dying at Murray Manor. New York: St. Martin's Press. 221 Pp.

The author used participant-observation for several months in 1973 to study Murray Manor. He served the nursing home in a number of capacities while making his observations, including work as a nursing assistant (at least to the extent of toileting residents) and as a gerontologist consultant at staff meetings. His objectives were to understand how the various participants in the home--staff and residents--negotiated their roles, goals, and needs; how they constructed their rights and duties; and how in the end, Murray Manor developed as an organized social entity. Most of its contents are highly relevant to the nursing assistant, especially chapters 4, 5, and 6: Body and Bed Work, Passing Time, and Death and Dying.

56. Kane, R., and Kane R. (1987). Long-term care. New York: Springer. 432 Pp.

This book provides an overview of current long-term care systems for the elderly. Extensive data about nursing home care, day care, foster care, respite care, and care management are pulled together. Moreover, the organization, function, and effects of these systems on their clients are assessed.

57. Kramer, C. H., and Kramer, J. R. (1976). Basic principles of long-term patient care: Developing a therapeutic community. Springfield, Ill.: Charles C. Thomas. 375 Pp.

This book applies aspects of organizational and family systems theories to the development of a therapeutic nursing home milieu. Particular attention is given to interpersonal relationships, communication, organizing the milieu, the special contribution of the nursing staff, resolving conflicts among the staff, and integrating services.

58. Preston, R. P. (1979). The dilemmas of care: Social and nursing adaptations to the deformed, the disabled and the aged. New York: Elsevier. 220 Pp.

This book is divided into two parts. The first part discusses the significance of "ambiguous persons," for example, the disabled, deformed, and the aged, and their challenge to their caretakers. The challenge and threat come from the clear mortality of the ambiguous persons, which is also a threat to the mortality of the caretakers. The second part of the book applies the ideas developed in the first half to a nursing staff in a community hospital. Many of the author's ideas emerged from his work as an LPN with this hospital for over six years. In the final chapter, the author outlines an approach for improving the humanitarian milieu of hospitals.

59. Price, J. L. (1977). The study of turnover. Ames: The Iowa State University Press. 160 Pp.

This intensive analysis of the literature (304 citations) on published turnover research since 1900 includes data from the United States as well as other Western societies. The review suggested the following determinants of turnover in a variety of occupations:

Successively lower amounts of pay will probably produce successively higher rates of turnover.

Successively lower degrees of organizational integration will probably produce higher amounts of turnover.

Successively lower amounts of formal and instrumental communication will probably produce successively higher amounts of turnover.

Successively higher degrees of centralization of power will probably produce successively higher amounts of turnover.

The research also found five correlates associated with turnover.

Personnel with short lengths of service usually have higher rates of turnover than those with long lengths of service.

Younger persons usually have higher rates of turnover than older persons.

During periods of high employment, there are usually higher rates of turnover than during periods of low employment.

Unskilled blue-collar workers usually have higher rates of turnover than skilled blue-collar workers.

Blue-collar workers usually have higher rates of turnover than white-collar workers.

60. Sherwood, S. (editor) (1975). Long-term care: A handbook for researchers, planners, and providers. New York: Spectrum. 788 Pp.

This comprehensive handbook contains thirteen chapters on the various aspects of long-term care ranging from psychosocial intervention programs within an institutional setting to the economic perspective of long-term care. The individual chapters are original pieces written by experts in the topics under consideration.

61. Stryker, R. (1981). How to reduce employee turnover in nursing homes and other health care organizations. Springfield, Ill.: Charles C. Thomas. 224 Pp.

This research studied the staff turnover in 110 Minnesota nursing homes. Data were generated on the total staff including nursing assistants, and the facilities. The sample represented 25 percent of the total number of nursing homes in the state. Two questionnaires, one on the characteristics of the facility and one on the characteristics of the administrators, were sent to the facilities sampled. A number of the conclusions were drawn from the study. The turnover rates were extremely variable and lower than expected. Of the 110 homes studied, only 10 had a high turnover rate for the total number of employees, and 22 had a high turnover rate for nursing assistants. The level of turnover was defined by the study (high: 81 percent or higher). Other findings, for both total number of employees and nursing assistants, included lower turnover in nursing homes located in small communities; in government supported nursing homes in contrast to proprietary homes; and in homes with fewer than seventy-five employees. When the turnover of only nursing assistants was considered, the rates were lower in facilities having less than 100 beds, and in homes having twenty-nine or fewer nursing assistants. Salary, presence of unions, and number of orientation days for newly employed nursing assistants were not significantly related to turnover, nor were any of the administrator's characteristics.

62.   Taylor, J. C., and Bowers, D. G. (1972). Survey of organizations. Ann Arbor: University of Michigan Press. 165 Pp.

This monograph reports the development of a standardized questionnaire to understand organizational conditions and practices. Though developed primarily for industry and business organizations, the latest edition of the questionnaire is for more general use. Two-thirds of its 105 items ask about the respondent's perceptions of the "organizational reality" that he or she has experienced in the recent past; the remaining third of the questions ask for reactions, feelings, desires, and dissatisfactions.

63.   Tobin, S. S., and Lieberman, M. A. (1976). Last home for the aged. San Francisco: Jossey-Bass. 304 Pp.

This research report describes how placing the elderly in nursing homes institutionalizes them. Prior to admission, the elderly are encouraged to think of becoming residents in nursing homes, and this concept is reinforced when the elderly enter a facility. Evaluating a sample of 100, the research investigated the effects of the decision to seek institutional care, of the first two months after entering, and after one year of living in an institution. Employing measures of cognitive functioning, affective responsiveness, emotional states, and self-perceptions, the research showed the greatest psychological damage occurred before entrance to the institution. However, the disruption of being placed into a nursing home, the enforced passivity, and being perceived as being unable to care for themselves also contributed to elderly people's loss of hope and despondence. Services to prevent premature institutionalization of persons entering nursing homes are suggested.

64.   U.S. Department of Health, Education, and Welfare, Public Health Service (1975). Long-term care facility improvement study. DHEW Pub. No.(OS)76-50021. Washington, D.C.: U.S. Government Printing Office. 137 Pp.

This report focuses on the nation's skilled nursing homes. It provides information on the care provided, the health status of the residents, and the physical environment and managerial setting as they affect both the quality and the cost of skilled nursing care. Detail on the survey methodology used in the study is fully presented including the sample and how it was selected, how the survey instruments were developed, and the manner in which the data were analyzed. The findings included: 22 percent (62,886) of the 283,915 residents surveyed were mentally retarded or developmentally disabled; a great number of residents were dependent on the nursing staff for their daily living; pharmaceutical services were adequate while physician, rehabilitative, nursing, and social services were inadequate. Also, the health and safety of the environment were wanting. Training for all disciplines was lacking. Findings suggested: a total review of the survey certification procedures of nursing homes; nationwide training; credentialing; certification and licensure of all state surveyors; and a complete analysis of the entire fiscal reimbursement program of supporting long-term care facilities. Alternatives to institutional care such as home health care and day care were suggested.

65. Vladeck, B. C. (1980). Unloving care: The nursing home tragedy. New York: Basic Books. 305 Pp.

The topic of this report is how public policy has failed to provide high-quality care for persons in nursing homes and what must be done to correct its errors. The book is detailed, scholarly, historical, as well as current, and places nursing homes in the broad context of social welfare and medical care of the elderly. Its recommendations suggest providing: nursing home care to only those persons who clearly require such care; congregate housing that has housekeeping and laundry equipment, recreation, and health and social services for the relatively healthy elderly; and home health care for a substantial number of elderly who can remain in the community. Policy recommendations of lesser scope suggest: improved nursing care, including psychosocial care, and housekeeping services in nursing homes. This report also describes the exceptionally difficult job of the nursing assistant.

66. York, J. L. (1977). Community mental health centers and nursing homes: Guidelines for cooperative programs. Lansing, Mich.: St. Lawrence Hospital, Community Mental Health Center. 105 Pp.

This is a manual to develop a cooperative program between community mental health centers and nursing homes. Specific directions cover the pertinent points to organize a program, including how to form a planning group, formulate written agreements, use case consultation, and proceed with staff training and program development. Sample forms to facilitate these developments are included.

JOURNALS

67. Aiken, L. H., Mezey, M. D., Lynaugh, J. E., and Buck, C. R. (1985). "Teaching nursing homes: Prospects for improving long-term care." Journal of the American Geriatrics Society, 33(3):196-201.

Strengthening the clinical services in nursing homes by implementing a concept of teaching nursing homes is presented. University nursing schools are well positioned to develop a teaching and consulting relationship with nursing homes to realize the teaching nursing home model. The major objective is to change the nature of care in nursing homes and thereby improve patient outcomes. Supplemental costs of creating a teaching nursing home are discussed. The clinical management skills of the additional staff could prevent unnecessary hospitalization of residents and encourage the admission of severely impaired, unstable, and disruptive patients who are currently turned away.

68. Barney, J. L. (1974). "Community presence as a key to quality of life in nursing homes." American Journal of Public Health, 64(3):265-268.

Direct community involvement and responsibility in the operation of nursing homes is proposed as a mechanism for improving the standards of nursing home care. The author recommends that each nursing home should be required by law to have an official board composed of residents, relatives, staff, and interested citizens. It would act as a protector, advocate, and friend of the residents, many of whom are without attentive families, and it would develop community contacts for the nursing home.

69. Bayer, M., Bresloff, L., and Curley, D. (1986). "The enhancement project." Geriatric Nursing, 7(4):192-195.

This project helped certified nursing assistants better meet the psychosocial needs of residents. Staff development included inservice training and opportunities for job advancement and improved level of practice. The project and its evaluation are set forth in qualitative terms.

70. Bennett, R. (1963). "The meaning of institutional life." The Gerontologist, 3(3):117-125.

The author used participant observation, content analysis, and interviewing over a period of five years to study the "Home" (a nonproprietary nursing home in New York City). Descriptions of its social structure; socialization of new residents; and the generation of meaning for administrators, professional staff, and residents are provided. The article also develops a typology of nursing homes using the extent to which a home controls the lives of its residents. The typology of high, medium, and low control is used to view the orientation and scheduling of activities, dissemination of normative information, institution's sanctions, and involvement of residents in decisionmaking.

71. Braden, B., Smith, C., and Bergstrom, N. (1988). "Paving the way to research in nursing homes." Geriatric Nursing, 9(1):38-41.

Guidelines are presented and discussed to encourage research in nursing homes. Particular attention is given to initiatives that ought to be taken by both the director of nursing and the researchers (outside the home) in developing and maintaining a research relationship.

72. Braun, J. V., Wykle, M. H., and Cowling, W. R. (1988). "Failure to thrive in older persons: A concept derived." The Gerontologist, 28(6):809-812.

The concept "failure to thrive," borrowed from pediatrics, is redefined for use in caring for the elderly. The concept is related to the austerity of the elderly person's environment.

73. Brody, E. M. (1973). "A million procrustean beds." The Gerontologist, 13(4):430-435.

This article argues for a new model of nursing home, one that would be developed from the residents' needs in the light of available knowledge. Resident options, choices, and respect are urged.

74. Carter, R., et al. (1988). "Importance of perceived values in nursing homes management." The Journal of Long-Term Care Administration, 16(2):10-13.

This study focuses on the turnover of nursing assistants as a consequence of inaccurate perceptions by nursing home administrators. The authors urge supportive communication, participation, and interpersonal relationships between supervisors and employees as ways to reduce turnover and improve organizational stability.

75. Cassel, C. K. (1988). "Ethical issues in the conduct of research in long-term care." The Gerontologist, 28(supplement):90-96.

Guidelines are presented emphasizing the appropriate setting and context of review for research in long-term care, clinical assessment of the residents' capacity to make decisions including giving informed consent to participate in research, and nursing home procedures to minimize any conflict of interest between the residents' need for care and the research interests.

76. Chekryn, J., and Roos, L. L. (1979). "Auditing the process of care in a new geriatric unit." Journal of the American Geriatrics Society, 27(3):107-111.

This project studied the extent to which a new geriatric unit met its objectives by assessing the residents' records. The study sampled 101 geriatric patients who were admitted to the unit for rehabilitative therapy. The study did not show a significant correlation between recorded care processes and treatment outcomes; however, it did show the extent to which care was provided.

77. Chenitz, W. C. (1983). "The nurse's aide and the confused person." Geriatric Nursing, 4(4):238-241.

The challenge of the confused resident to the nursing assistant and techniques to care for her are presented. Also, the nursing assistant's efforts to generate personal meanings from such work are considered. The nursing assistant's positive relationships to the resident, and to peers, nurses, and employer are suggested as the resident, and to peers, nurses, and employer are suggested as the best way of generating personal meanings. Encouragement to the nursing assistant is advised.

78. Feder, J., and Scanlon, W. (1980). "Regulating the bed supply in nursing homes." Milbank Memorial Fund Quarterly, 58(1):54-88.

Expenditures for nursing home care are large. For example, they made up 29 percent of the Medicaid budget in 1977. Faced with this fiscal demand in the 1970s, many states took measures to limit their liabilities. This article analyzed the states' measures to restrict the bed supply in nursing homes through "certification-of-need" regulation. The authors argue that the regulation of the bed supply exacerbated rather than eliminated inefficiencies in the market for long-term care. They concluded that, if expenditure control is to be compatible with efficient and equitable allocation of resources, the states must use their payment to ensure more certainly that care is available to the persons who need it most.

79. Goldfarb, A. I. (1953). "Recommendations for psychiatric care in a home for the aged." Journal of Gerontology, 8(3):343-347.

After three years of employing a psychiatrist in a nursing home it was decided by the nurses and social workers engaged in the project (along with the half-time participating psychiatrist) that a full-time psychiatrist would be helpful. The investigation-trial period included having the psychiatrist involved in the diagnostic examination of the residents, education of the staff, the screening of job applicants, and individual and group psychotherapy. Longer-term possibilities at the nursing home included: the development of psychotherapeutic techniques, the enhancement of the milieu for therapeutic purposes, and the improvement of procedures to evaluate applicants for admission to nursing home care.

80. Gottesman, L. E. (1970). "Organizing rehabilitation services for the elderly." The Gerontologist, 10(4):287-293.

Nursing homes provide mostly physical care and medical rehabilitative services and neglect psychosocial needs. Strategies for reorganization must take account of the characteristics of the nursing home, residents, staff, and the administrator. Of these, the selection and training of the administrator is suggested as being the

81. Gottesman, L. E. (1973). "Milieu treatment of aged in institutions." The Gerontologist, 13(1):23-26.

This article reflects the importance of the nursing home environment--staff attitudes and initiatives, administrative style and support, the daily interactions between the staff, the relations among the staff and residents, and the staff's willingness to change.

82. Grant, N. K., and Hrycak, N. (1987). "Use of the critical incident technique to elicit the opinions of residents of long-term-care facilities about their care." Nursing Homes, 36(3):38-44.

The critical incident technique was used to get information on eighteen categories of service in three nursing homes and three auxiliary hospitals. Only four of the categories are reported on: information given before admission, responses about settling into a new environment, nursing care, and provision of privacy. The subjects were 409 residents selected by the director of nursing or her delegate. They were physically capable of hearing and speaking English and were believed to be capable of answering the questions. A substantial number of responses indicated difficulties in getting settled in a nursing home, lack of useful information before admission, and lack of privacy. Also, negative responses were registered about nursing care. No statistical analysis other than arranging the basic data was provided.

83. Gustafson, D., Fiss, C., Fryback, J., Smelser, P., and Hiles, M. (1981). "Quality of care in nursing homes: The new Wisconsin evaluation system." The Journal of Long-Term Care Administration, 9(2):40-55.

Procedures to evaluate the quality of nursing home care were set forth, including forms to be completed by members of the assessment team (nurse, social worker, sanitarian, and administrator). These were designed to overcome the shortcomings of the traditional evaluation procedures required to participate in the Medicaid program. The criticisms of the traditional evaluation procedures were their inflexibility, inefficient allocation of time and resources, and inability to bring about changes.

84. Gutman, G. M., and Herbert, C. P. (1976). "Mortality rates among
     relocated extended-care patients." Journal of Gerontology,
     31(3):352-357.

     Eighty-one male extended-care patients, relocated due to
     demolition of their building, were followed for twenty-one months
     from the date of their transfer. No increase in the mortality rate
     was observed during the first three months of the postrelocation
     period, an interval usually associated with high mortality of elderly
     persons involuntarily relocated. During the first year after
     relocation, the death rate was 33.33 percent compared to an
     average annual death rate of 41.20 percent at the facility during the
     preceding five years. At twenty-one months half of the relocated
     population were still alive. These data contrast with previous
     studies, most of which indicated increased mortality after
     relocation. The article suggests a number of important factors in
     the relocation of elderly residents: careful preparation of residents,
     limited disruption of daily routines, family visitation, increased
     visitation by attending physicians, and active support by nursing
     staff.

85. Hansing, L. (1986). "A program for the emotionally disturbed."
     Geriatric Nursing, 7(3):137-139.

     The background and current status of special units in a
     Minneapolis hospital for aged persons who are emotionally
     disturbed are presented. The milieu and special treatment efforts
     and some patient outcomes are described.

86. Harris, A., and Chermak, J. B. (1987). "PCAs: Hillhaven's career
     ladder option." Provider, 13(4):32-34.

     The patient care assistant program developed by the Hillhaven
     Corporation includes three levels of patient care assistants.
     Further, persons reaching the third level are encouraged to
     continue their progression by entering professional nurse's training
     with corporate scholarship support. Leadership training was given
     to all supervising nurses and department heads on the details of
     the program before it was initiated. Increased salaries, new job
     titles and duties, and graduation ceremonies are linked to each
     rung in the career ladder.

87. Hoch, C., and Reynolds, C. (1986). "Sleep disturbances and what
to do about them." Geriatric Nursing, 7(1):24-27.

Causal factors for sleep disturbances are presented and a number
of measures to improve sleep are suggested. Sleep disturbances
among the elderly, while common, are not trivial. Residents may
have a number of complaints in addition to their sleeping
disturbances, when such disturbances are concurrent with medical
or psychiatric disorders and environmental changes.

88. Houghton, J. G. (1965). "Organization of medical services in a
private nursing home--three new approaches." New England
Journal of Medicine, 272(19):996-1003.

The recent history of proprietary nursing homes in New York City
is reviewed, and the nursing home population of the city is
described. Three approaches to the organization of medical
services in nursing homes are discussed and some experiences
reported. Briefly, the three approaches are: (1) prepayment
mechanism in purchasing medical services for recipients of public
assistance; (2) a hospital-assigned medical staff under the
supervision of the clinical coordinator providing medical care to
the nursing home; and (3) using the services of physicians in the
community. The advantages and problems of these approaches are
discussed.

89. Hughes, D. C., and Peters, G. R. (1978). "Organizational position
and perceptions of problems in a nursing home." Journal of
Gerontology, 33(2):279-287.

Data from administrative staff, professional and nonprofessional
nursing staffs, therapy staff, auxiliary staff, and residents, generated
through interview observations and analyses of records, indicated
that organizational position was related to the perception of
nursing home problems.

90. Ingram, D. K., and Barry, J. R. (1977). "National statistics on
deaths in nursing homes." The Gerontologist, 17(4):303-308.

National statistics for three data periods over a ten-year span are
presented to show the increasing numbers of elderly who are dying
in nursing homes. Several statistical indexes are presented to
describe this trend. This phenomenon underscores the need for

more extensive orientation of nursing home personnel on managing death.

91. Jones, D. C. (1975). "Special proximity, interpersonal conflict, and friendship formation in the intermediate care facility." The Gerontologist, 15(2):150-154.

In this study of 441 residents in ten nursing homes it was found that close proximity did not necessarily produce positive relations. Interpersonal conflict was found to occur more often between residents residing within a distance of two rooms. Those residents who lived at a greater distance from each other were better able to maintain positive relations.

92. Kane, R. L., Bell, R., Riegler, S., Wilson, A., and Keeler, E. (1983). "Predicting the outcomes of nursing home patients." The Gerontologist, 23(2):202-206.

This article proposes a system of nursing home reimbursement based on attaining achievable objectives. Using three waves of data collected at three-month intervals on approximately 250 patients, the authors were able to predict patient functioning in six areas (physiologic, activities, affective, cognitive, social and personal satisfaction). However, their predictions of discharge (better, worse, or dead) were less accurate. An instrument was developed to obtain data from patients by testing their performance and by interviewing them.

93. Kane, R. L., and Kane, R. A. (1980). "Long-term care versus tender loving care." In Williams, S. J., and Torrens, P. R. (editors). Introduction to health services. New York: John Wiley & Sons, 508 Pp.

This chapter provides an overview of long-term care. The term implies a distinction from the acute services available in the hospital and physicians' offices. It indicates the dependence of an individual on the services of another for a substantial period (and not necessarily medical services). The service may be provided by family, friends, or neighbors. This chapter addresses five major questions: (1) Why is long-term care an issue? (2) Who is at risk? (3) What is the role of the nursing home? (4) How did we get to where we are? (5) What can be done about it?

94. Kane, R. L., and Kane, R. A. (1980). "The nursing home: Neither home nor hospital." In Williams, S. J., and Torrens, P. R. (editors). Introduction to health services. New York: John Wiley and Sons, 508 Pp.

This material considers the long-term care needs of society with a particular emphasis on the role of nursing homes. It emphasizes the social and environmental concerns that must be considered by any examination of services, and notes the failure to maintain this broad perspective. The chapter reviews the historical development of nursing homes, provides descriptive data on their character, considers the problem of paying for nursing home care, sets forth the character of medical services to residents, and describes the low quality of life in nursing homes. It also considers the differences between medical and social models of nursing homes. Overall it advocates that institutions for the elderly, whether they are called nursing homes or old age homes, should be developed as dwelling places for those elderly who are most likely to have serious and chronic health problems.

95. Kaplan, J., and Ford, C. S. (1975). "Rehabilitation for the elderly: An eleven-year assessment." The Gerontologist, 5(4):393-397.

One thousand one hundred thirty-five discharged geriatric patients (aged sixty-two through ninety-nine) from the rehabilitation service in a skilled nursing home during the period 1963 through 1974 served as the subjects for the evaluation study. They had received medical attention, occupational therapy, social work services, and speech therapy. Six hundred ninety-three, or 61 percent, of discharged residents returned to independent living in their own households. This percent of return was attributed to a comprehensive health team approach, including high quality physical care and social work consultation in the nursing home and social work assistance in the placement of residents.

96. Keeler, E. B., Kane, R. L., and Soloman, D. H. (1981). "Short- and long-term residents of nursing homes." Medical Care, 19(3):363-369.

This article presents an analysis of the residents' length of stay in nursing homes. Data was drawn from the 1977 National Nursing Home Survey. The analysis indicated there were two separate streams of populations passing through the nursing homes: a

short-stay group whose average length of stay was approximately
1.8 months and a long-stay group who stayed about 2.5 years.

97. Kelman, H. R., and Muller, J. N. (1962).   "Rehabilitation of
     nursing home residents." Geriatrics, 17(6):402-411.

This research studied matched samples of randomly assigned
treated and untreated disabled public-assistance-supported nursing
home residents. The change criteria, including levels of functioning
in ambulation, dressing, and feeding and toileting skills, indicated
a low rate of rehabilitation.

98. Knapp, M., and Harissis, K. (1981). "Staff vacancies and turnover
     in British old people's homes." The Gerontologist, 21(1):76-84.

The high rate of domestic staff vacancies and turnover, low rates
of recruitment, and shortages of suitably qualified or skilled
candidates have long troubled the British old people's homes. A
framework for research and policy for these problems is set forth
and some research findings are presented.   The framework
included: (1) characteristics of the job (pay, hours, promotion
opportunities, organization of tasks, home design, staff
accommodations, resident dependency, and services offered);
(2) characteristics of the individual (age, sex, marital status, basic
education, qualifications, and length of service); and (3) other
factors (labor markets and location of home). Research findings
from the 1970 Census of Residential Accommodation reported:
homes that offered a variety of services including meals for the
elderly living in the neighborhood had fewer domestic staff
problems than homes with the opposite pattern; domestic staff
vacancies were greatest in homes of poor design; homes that were
badly sited in relation to amenities for residents, such as shops,
churches, pubs, and transportation, had a considerable number of
domestic staff vacancies; and the greater the responsibility accorded
supervisory staff the more attractive the home was for the domestic
staff.

99. Kohn, G. L., and Biache, A. S. (1982). "Developing a career ladder
     for nursing personnel."   The Journal of Long-Term Care
     Administration, 10(4):25-27.

This is a description of a nursing home's career ladder for its
nursing assistants. Aimed at curbing its high rate of job turnover,

and to fill gaps in the home's services, steps in the ladder included:

Senior nursing assistant was the first step up. Persons selected for this position had to be reliable, compassionate, take the initiative in their work, work cooperatively with their supervisors, and be dedicated to the role of a nursing assistant. A special emblem was given to them for wearing on the left sleeve as a visible sign of their status.

Ward clerk and personal care coordinator were the second step up. These positions did not require direct bedside care.

A licensed practical nurse was the last step up.

In addition, the program encouraged additional education for RNs and licensed practical nurses. A qualitative assessment of the program indicated the career ladder generated loyalty among the staff, decreased turnover, brought fresh approaches to the nursing home, and improved the residents' level of care.

100. Kosberg, J. I. (1974). "Making institutions accountable: Research and policy issues." The Gerontologist, 14(6):510-516.

This article organizes its discussion of accountability around two major questions: accountability of what? accountability to whom? It concludes that research will guide policy of reimbursement that rewards and provides incentives for restorative care. The article also recommends an active role for physicians and their organizations in nursing homes, and suggests that professionals employed within institutions are no less professional than their colleagues in noninstitutional settings.

101. Lawton, M. P. (1970). "Institutions for the aged: Theory, content, and methods for research." The Gerontologist, 10(4):305-312.

This article traces the implications of organizational systems theory for the study of nursing homes. The following components of the theory are given detailed consideration: (1) the production system, whose goal is technical proficiency; (2) the maintenance system, which strives for organizational stability; (3) the boundary system, which is concerned with procuring residents and manipulating the facility environment to maintain a smooth flow of care and treatment activities; (4) the adaptive system, which is focused on planning and effecting organizational changes in response to community demands; and (5) the managerial system, which is aimed at preserving or improving the nursing home by coordinating the several systems of the facility and their community relationships. The article concludes with suggestions about research methods that might be used in studying nursing homes: cataloging the many variables of the facility that pertain to the systems, using factor analysis to reduce them to smaller sets and thereby producing a taxonomy; intercorrelating the items obtained for each system to generate information about their relationships; and using this knowledge to mount more sophisticated evaluation studies of nursing homes.

102. Lawton, M. P., Patnaik, B., and Kleban, M. H. (1976). "The ecology of adaptation to a new environment." International Journal of Aging and Human Development, 7(1):15-26.

Behavior mapping techniques were used to study the effects of transferring forty-eight elderly residents from one room to another in a nursing home. Data were obtained on the physical location, body position, and behavior of residents on their residential floors preceding and following the transfer. Among the findings were the resident's strong increase in passive behavior following transfer. This was interpreted as the residents' taking time to reestablish their orientation to their physical and social surroundings and reconstituting their resources for more actively dealing with their environment in the future.

103. Lee, Y. S. (1984). "Nursing homes and quality of health care: The first year result of an outcome-oriented survey." Journal of the Health and Human Resources Administration (JHHRA), 7(1):32-60.

Using information gathered by an "outcome-oriented" licensure survey, this article concluded that Iowa satisfactorily met the requirement for nursing and personal care services, and provided clean and well-maintained living environments. However, the nursing homes performed poorly in care planning and review and implementing the physicians' orders on medication, treatment, and diet schedules. The nursing facilities for nonprofit provided better quality care than the facilities for profit, and small proprietary facilities performed consistently poorer than large facilities, especially large nonprofit-oriented facilities.

104. Lieberman, M. A. (1969). "Institutionalization of the aged: Effects on behavior." Journal of Gerontology, 24(3):330-340.

This article reviews the literature on how being institutionalized effects the behavior of elderly persons. Studies of geriatric centers, nursing homes, domiciliaries, and chronic disease units are included as well as facilities that serve a larger number of aged but are not exclusively oriented toward them, such as mental hospitals. Also, the article sets forth future research, particularly as it might influence policy development.

105. Linn, M. W. (1966). "A nursing home rating scale." Geriatrics, 21(10):188-192.

The suggested rating scale provides a means of determining which nursing homes are more likely to provide good care, although further efforts are needed to assess properly the ultimate effectiveness of such facilities.

106. Linn, M. W. (1967). "A rapid disability rating scale." Journal of the American Geriatric Society, 15(2):211-214.

Rapid Disability Rating Scale (PDRS) contains sixteen items (on eating, diet, medication, speech, learning, sight, walking, bathing, dressing, incontinence, shaving, safety supervision, confinement to bed, mental confusion, uncooperation, and depression). Items have a three-point frequency of occurrence. The scale is primarily a technique for assessing treatment changes, and for use in research on chronic illness. However, its use may be extended to screening for care and for ward classification. The scale is highly reliable and valid.

107. Linn, M. W., Gurel, L., and Linn, B. S. (1977). "Patient outcome as a measure of quality of nursing home care." American Journal of Public Health, 67(4):337-344.

Over a nine-year period, male patients placed from a general medical Veterans' Administration hospital in Miami were studied immediately before transfer to community nursing homes, one week after transfer, and six months later. Demographic information, health data, physician's prediction of patient's condition if six months of optimal nursing home care were provided (improvement, deterioration, or no change) and ward nurse evaluation of each patient were collected. The patients' outcomes were related to the nursing home characteristics by multivariate analysis controlling for expected outcome, age, and diagnoses of cancer and chronic brain disease. Nursing homes with more RN hours per patient were associated with patients being alive, improved, and discharged from the homes. Better ratings on the quality of the nursing homes' food service were positively associated with the patients being alive and improved. Also, higher professional staff-to-patient ratio, better medical records, and more services were related to being discharged from nursing homes. The more elusive, yet important, phenomena of nursing homes such as their psychosocial "atmosphere" and personalities of their staff members were recognized by the study, but not pursued.

108. McClanahan, L. E. (1973). "Therapeutic and prosthetic living environments for nursing home residents." The Gerontologist, 13(4):424-429.

Environmental variables thought to impact on the residents of nursing homes were drawn from the literature and explored in depth. The variables of greatest concern were those that seemingly had some effect on the locomotion, interaction, and self-care skills of the elderly. Proposals were made for the types of research that might contribute to developing nursing home environments that encourage and maintain the desired behavior and retard the degenerative processes associated with aging.

109. McClanahan, L. E., and Risley, T. R. (1974). "Design of living environments for nursing home residents: Recruiting attendance at activities." The Gerontologist, 14(3):236-240.

Announcements for recruiting attendance at activities-- announcements over the house public address system, and large-print signs placed at the entrance to the dining hall--were tested for their effectiveness in bringing residents to activities. Data demonstrated that these announcements were effective in prompting high levels of attendance, and that failure to use them resulted in more than a 50 percent reduction in attendance.

110. McClanahan, L. E., and Risley, T. R. (1975). "Design of living environments for nursing home residents: Increasing participation in recreation activities." Journal of Applied Behavior Analysis, 8(3):261-268.

This study examined the residents' participation in the lounge area of a nursing home. Attendance in the lounge varied greatly, depending on the availability of materials, and the method of making them available. The research indicated that the engagement of the residents could be trebled by providing manipulative materials (for example, games and puzzles) and prompting residents to use them. Further, the study demonstrated that prompting can effectively maintain the residents' participation with manipulating materials, and that merely making equipment available and waiting for residents to take the initiative in requesting and using it typically resulted in low levels of participation.

111. McGrowder-Lin, R., and Bhatt, A. (1988). "A wanderer's lounge program for nursing home residents with Alzheimer's disease." The Gerontologist, 28(4):607-609.

A wanderer's lounge serving fifteen to twenty residents was established to provide activities to benefit Alzheimer's victims, and allow respite for more alert residents and staff on the living units. The wanderer's lounge sought to sustain the residents' interpersonal relationships, maintain their dignity, and avoid dependency. The attitude of the caregivers was one of friendliness and caring. Nursing assistants interrupted aggressive behavior by directing the residents' attention or distracting them. Techniques included starting a sing-a-long or spontaneous dancing sessions. The benefits of the lounge are discussed from a qualitative perspective.

112. McGuire, H. (1975). "New laws and regulations must focus on continuity of care." Hospital, 49(10):63-67.

This article suggests drafters of laws and regulations should attend to past failures and inadequacies: restrictive regulations or interpretations of them, uneven and sometimes heavy-handed administration of the regulations (for example, preoccupation with costs to the detriment of residents needs), and the inappropriateness and poor quality of care.

113. Meer, B., and Baker, J. A. (1966). "The Stockton geriatric rating scale." Journal of Gerontology, 21(3):392-403.

This scale focuses on four behavioral factors: physical disability, apathy, communication failure, and socially irritating behavior. Although intercorrelated, these factors measure somewhat different aspects of the geriatric resident's daily behavior in a facility. The scale's reliability and validity are presented as adequate.

114. Miller, D. B. (1975). "Sexual practices and administrative policies in long-term care institutions." The Journal of Long-Term Care Administration, 3(3):30-40.

Issues facing the administration of long-term care institutions governing sexual behavior by the residents are discussed, and a number of alternative policies are offered. Though focused on the facility's administration, the article has direct relevance for nursing assistants who would be involved in the implementation of any policy, for example, in managing the facility's physical environment and in facilitating or restricting sexual contact between various kinds of couples, and solo sexual activity.

115. Miller, M. B. (1975). "Iatrogenic and nursigenic effects of prolonged immobilization of the ill aged." Journal of the American Geriatrics Society, 23(8):360-369.

The physician-induced and nurse-induced immobilization of the ill aged has psychological, psychosocial, physiological, and biochemical effects. Factors related to such disabilities are described and illustrated. These conditions are viewed as being reversible.

116. Mitchell, J. B. (1978). "Patient outcomes in alternative long-term care settings." Medical Care, 16(6):439-452.

Health status outcomes are compared in three Veterans' Administration alternative long-term care settings: (1) home care, (2) community-based nursing home care, and (3) hospital-based nursing home care. Patients had their health measured on a behavioral index when they were transferred from an acute care hospital to one of the three treatment programs, and again three months later. Patients were not randomly distributed to the programs; two research methods were employed to reduce sample selection bias: a nonequivalent control group was chosen and multivariate analytic statistical procedures were used. Further, within each program type, the patients were randomly selected from both a hospital that offered only that program as a long-term care alternative and from a hospital that provided all three treatment settings. Patients placed in the home care program displayed the greatest mean improvement in their health; however, this effect was not uniform as patients showed different rates of improvement across the three programs, based upon their initial health status and prognosis.

117. Morris, R. (1966). "Expansion of cooperative relationships between hospitals and nursing homes." Public Health Reports, 75(12):110-114.

Five major types of cooperation--informal arrangements for patient transfer, training exchanges, joint program planning, joint appointment of key staff, and administrative integration--indicate several ways by which hospital and nursing home relations can be strengthened to enhance patient care and community health planning.

118. Morrow-Winn, G. (1985). "When the pressures mount: Recognizing and coping with stress." Nursing Homes, 34(1):39-42.

This essay considers nursing home employees' response to societal and work stress. Management and personal actions to prevent and ameliorate stress are provided. Among the pointers to management are: increase communication to all employees, especially when any change is to occur; introduce and orient new personnel; make sure new personnel have the knowledge and skill to do their jobs; balance the care load of personnel so it has a mix of easy to care for residents with hard-to-care-for ones; encourage employees to communicate their concerns; evaluate alternative ways to schedule and assign work; and design staff development programs that help staff identify, prevent, and cope with work-related stress. Suggestions to individual staff members include: learn to read signals of stress in oneself; develop a sense of self that is not dependent on others; and acquire coping skills to deal with symptoms of stress.

119. Noelker, L., and Harel, Z. (1978). "Predictors of well-being and survival among institutionalized aged." The Gerontologist, 18(6):562-567.

This study sought to ascertain predictors of the well-being and survival among the less-impaired older residents who relocate voluntarily into what they consider to be a better environment, and who can maintain control over that environment. Analysis of initial interviews and two-year followup data showed that primary predictors of morale, life satisfaction, satisfaction with treatment, and survival were the residents' subjective perceptions of the facility and their preference to live in it. The findings also indicated more careful attention must be given to the residents' cognitive and emotional states at several points--time of application, entering into the new location, and throughout their stay--to help them with their well-being and survival.

120. Norville, J. L., and Breindel, C. L. (1981). "Monitoring departmental performance in the long-term care facility." The Journal of Long-Term Care Administration, 9(2):29-40.

This article describes the concept of an ongoing operational audit program, and its procedures to estimate the effectiveness and efficiency of various aspects of a nursing home program. Illustrations of its steps and procedures are provided.

121. Ohta, R. J., and Ohta, B. M. (1988). "Special units for Alzheimer's disease patients: A critical look." The Gerontologist, 28(6):803-808.

A review of special units for nursing home residents with senile dementia of the Alzheimer's type was provided. Published and unpublished reports, policy manuals, and personal observations were considered. The critical aspects of the units were identified and differences among the units were noted. Particular issues requiring the attention of researchers and program planners were discussed.

122. Pecarchick, R., and Nelson, B. H. (1973). "Employee turnover in nursing homes." American Journal of Nursing, 73(2):289-290.

A study of thirty-two nonprofit and fifty-one proprietary nursing homes in Pennsylvania compared turnover with salaries and fringe benefits of staff and services and facilities for residents. Turnover of nursing assistants was higher in proprietary than in nonprofit ones. However, turnover was also a problem in some of the nonprofit homes. Lower salaries, fewer fringe benefits, and more limited services and facilities to residents accounted for the differences in turnover in the two types of facilities.

123. Perlberg, M. (1979). "It works better when problems are shared."
     Hospitals, 53(1):70-74.

     This article reports an exclusive interview by the author with
     Jeannette R. Kramer, a specialist in the provision of long-term
     care, on the concept of the therapeutic community. One of the
     features of such a community is an environment in which patients,
     their families, and the staff can communicate easily and openly.
     That feature is the major theme of the interview. The openness
     allows various persons to contribute to the patients' care, and
     identify problems early on, at a point when they can be solved
     more easily.

124. Pinder, M. M. (1981). "Achievement of desired effects among
     nursing homes." The Journal of Long-Term Care Administration,
     9(2):56-61.

     This paper is concerned with the deleterious effects of
     institutionalization and suggests innovation and risking failure must
     be substituted for clinging to tradition and the known. Other
     suggestions include viewing the nursing home as a field of inquiry.
     The administrator is urged to solicit ideas from staff, residents,
     families, and the community.

125. Plutchik, R., Conte, H., Lieberman, M., Bakur, M., Grossman, J.,
     and Liehrman, N. (1970). "Reliability and validity of a scale for
     assessing the functioning of geriatric patients." Journal of the
     American Geriatrics Society, 18(6):491-500.

     A simple, objective rating scale for geriatric patients was developed
     and used to evaluate a sample of 207 patients at Bronx State
     Hospital for their physical and psychosocial functioning.
     Evaluations were made mainly by nursing assistants. The thirty-
     item scale, which has a three-point range for each item (never,
     sometimes, and often) had a high interjudge reliability and a high
     validity checked against clinical rating of patients by psychiatrists.

126. Powell, R. R. (1974). "Psychological effects of exercise therapy
     upon institutionalized geriatric mental patients." Journal of
     Gerontology, 29(2):157-161.

     This article reports an effort to influence certain cognitive and
     behavioral characteristics of institutionalized geriatric mental

patients with exercise therapy. Thirteen male and seventeen female geriatric patients were divided into two therapy groups (social therapy and exercise therapy) and one control group in a randomized block design that accounted for age, sex, and ward residence. Both forms of therapy were administered for twelve weeks. Three cognitive tests and two behavioral scales were used to evaluate all three groups prior to the treatment, after eight weeks of treatment, and at the completion of treatment (twelve weeks). Statistical analysis of variance indicated significant improvement in the cognitive skills of the persons who were exposed to the exercise therapy compared to those who received social therapy or received nothing. However, no significant differences were found in the behavioral skills of the three groups of patients as a result of the program.

127. Rantz, M., and Miller, T. V. (1983). "'Tailor-made' long term care." Nursing Management, 14(12):25-33.

Systematically recorded observations on such items as the provision of direct care to residents, making beds, cleaning activities, and formal and informal reporting on the condition of the residents were made on each nursing assistant in a large Midwestern skilled nursing home. The observations covered all ten nursing units and were made every fifteen seconds for thirty minutes. These data were categorized and quantified. Two work samples, each covering a twenty-four-hour period, were used for analysis. The numbers of nursing assistants on duty during the home's three shifts ranged from sixteen at night to forty-two in the day. Evaluation of the findings lead to reorganization of the facility that streamlined the lines of communication, responsibility, and accountability. Also, nonproductive activity was reduced. Questionnaires were used to evaluate the reorganization.

128. Reagan, J. T. (1986). "Management of nurse's aides in long-term care settings." The Journal of Long-Term Care Administration, 4(2):9-14.

Working from the literature on long-term care and experience in personnel administration, the author urged administrators of long-term care institutions to review their personnel management policies to ensure that all nursing assistants have the training, skill, and time required to perform their duties effectively and efficiently. The author also suggested that the administrators adopt policies and practices that will help solve and prevent problems unique to long-term care facilities. In addition, the author provided a format of detailed recommended actions for nursing facilities, their corporations, industrywide networks, and society-government entities to improve human resource management in long-term care.

129. Ryan, D. P., Tainish, S.M.M., Kolodny, V., Lendrum, B. L., and Fisher, R. H. (1988). "Noise-making amongst the elderly in long-term care." The Gerontologist, 28(3):369-371.

A typology of noise making was constructed: purposeless and perseverative noise-making, noise-making in response to the environment, noise-making to elicit a response from the environment, chatterbox noise-making, noise-making in the context of deafness, and other noise- making. One hundred twenty-two nursing staff were asked about the noise-making of 400 residents in a large metropolitan teaching hospital. The survey indicated that 30 percent of the residents engaged in noise-making. The clinical value of the typology and the findings of the survey were discussed.

130. Scanlon, W. J. (1980). "Nursing home utilization patterns." Journal of Health Politics, Policy and Law, 4(4):619-641.

This article reviews research on nursing home utilization with regard to several policy issues concerning the subsidization of long-term care by Medicaid, and indicates how Medicaid reimbursement and support and nursing home policies can result in a chronic shortage of beds. It also describes the dynamics of the policy by using eight variables: Medicaid generosity, age structure, family resources, racial composition, residence, financial capability of the elderly, price of nursing home care, and alternative sources of care. The article concludes that there is a need for: subsidization of a more comprehensive set of long-term care services, a review of reimbursement policies, and improved methods of allocating existing nursing home beds among persons desiring care.

131. Scanlon, W. J. (1980). "A theory of the nursing home market." Inquiry, 17(1):25-41.

Excessive demand for nursing home beds is generated by residents supported by private and public funds. Yet the market is segmented because Medicaid rates are too low to compete for the available beds. Problems of equity and efficiency emerge and are distinct from need. However, "need" has never been defined; this limits the analysis. In choosing among prospective residents, nursing homes are concerned about the costs of treating individual residents and, as a result, may discriminate against the most severely impaired. Medicaid funds recognize differences among states in their ability to fund the program and hence base each state's matching rate on its relative per capita income. However, there is a 50 percent ceiling on the state's rate. Elderly persons' ability to acquire long-term care, then, becomes a function of their geographic location rather than national criteria.

132. Scholz, R., and Brenner, G. (1977). "Relocation of the aged: A review and theoretical analysis." Journal of Gerontology, 32(3):323-333.

This article analyzes the literature on the relocation of the aged. Its findings are presented in terms of three types of moves-- institution to institution, home to institution, and home to home --with each type having a voluntary and involuntary component. A theoretical model is proposed to explain the often contradictory research findings. That model suggests that individuals respond to relocation in terms of the perceived predictability and controllability of the events surrounding the move, and the actual differences in the controllability of pre- and postrelocation environments. Suggestions are made for future study.

133. Silverstone, B., and Wynter, L. (1975). "The effects of introducing a heterosexual living space." The Gerontologist, 15(1):83-87.

Efforts to integrate the previously all male and female living units in a nursing home are reported. Several instruments are used to measure the effects of the integration, among them the Obleder Attitude Scale and the Ward Behavior Inventory. Quantitative and qualitative findings encouraged the authors to suggest the importance of heterosexual units particularly because they increase the interaction among the residents and enhance their sociability, particularly among the males.

134. Simmons, V., Fittipaldi, L., Holovet, E., Mones, P., Gerardi, R., and Mech, A. (1981). "Assessing the quality of care in skilled nursing homes." The Journal of Long-Term Care Administration, 9(2):1-28.

This article reports research to measure the quality of care in Maryland's skilled nursing homes. Four homes were drawn randomly from the state's list of skilled nursing homes. Both rural and urban, and proprietary and nonproprietary institutions were represented. Ninety residents were selected for their age, length of stay in the facility, and ability to perform specified activities of daily living. Of these, only fifty subjects or their families signed a consent to participate in the study. Observations were made daily between 8 a.m. and 2 p.m. Each observation lasted fifty-five minutes. Personnel observed included registered nurses, licensed practical nurses, and nursing assistants. Data were recorded on the Wandett Quality Patient Care Scale. Major findings were: (1) skilled nursing facilities located in urban areas provided a higher quality of care than did skilled nursing facilities located in rural areas, (2) nonproprietary skilled nursing homes provided a higher quality of care than proprietary skilled facilities, (3) a lower patient-staff ratio on living units increased the quality of care, (4) the quality of care improved as the number of licensed nursing personnel increased, (5) the quality of care improved when the ratio of residents requiring skilled care was lower than residents needing intermediate care, and (6) the quality of care increased as the number of support services increased.

135. Stannard, C. I. (1973). "Old folks and dirty work: The social conditions for patient abuse in a nursing home." Social Problems, 20(3):329-342.

Participant-observation-generated data on the abuse of residents in a nursing home suggested that the daily conditions of work keep the nurses from seeing or hearing about patient abuse. Further, these conditions also provide the nurses with routine ways to deny its occurrence when such a claim is made. These conditions include: the invisibility of nursing assistant-resident interactions, suspicion that separates the nurses from the rest of the employees, and distorted accounts of "what happened."

136. Stotsky, B. A. (1966). "Nursing homes: A review." The American Journal of Psychiatry, 123(3):249-258.

The history of nursing homes is presented. The areas of general medical care, rehabilitation, psychiatric evaluation, and therapy are emphasized. The concept of a custodial institution is rejected in favor of a rehabilitative institution; however, for homes to become rehabilitative depends on their ability to broaden and to professionalize their functions.

137. Stryker, R. S. (1982). "The effect of managerial interventions on high personnel turnover in nursing homes." Journal of Long-Term Care Administration, 10(2):21-26.

The findings of this research support the idea that turnover is related to many interrelated variables including training, orientation, ownership, location, size, supervision, pay, and benefits. Several procedures to reduce turnover were suggested: increased supervision of new employees, supervisory training, revised personnel policies, increased recruitment efforts, and avoiding use of personnel pools.

138. Teeter, R. B., Garetz, F. K., Miller, W. R., and Heiland, W. F. (1976). "Psychiatric disturbances of aged patients in skilled nursing homes." American Journal of Psychiatry, 133(12):1430-1434.

Research found that 85 percent of seventy-four residents supported by Medicaid in two skilled nursing facilities had significant psychiatric disorders in addition to serious multiple medical illnesses. Almost two-thirds of the psychiatric disturbances had not been diagnosed. Staff were more concerned with the psychosocial concerns of the residents than their physical concerns. Yet the staff had difficulty recognizing the legitimacy of one half of the residents' psychological complaints, and had difficulty relating to these residents. Also, the staff did not understand the physicians' orders for psychotropic medications. More psychiatric consultation was suggested to ensure appropriate and effective care of psychologically disturbed residents.

139. Tolbert, B. M. (1984). "Reality orientation and remotivation in a long-term care facility." Nursing and Health Care, 5(1):40-45.

This article describes a pilot program in reality orientation, attitude therapy, and remotivation of nursing home residents. Nursing assistants showed an increased awareness of the residents as persons with feelings, intellects, defenses, and wishes, as a result of the program. Also, the nursing assistants became increasingly more optimistic and hopeful about what the residents could accomplish and/or cope with. Though data were generated they had not been fully analyzed.

140. Trierweider, R. (1978). "Personal space and its effects on an elderly individual in a long-term care institution." Journal of Gerontological Nursing, 4(5):21-23.

This article emphasizes the importance of spatial and related arrangements to the well-being of residents in nursing homes. It recommends: (1) limiting size of institutions, (2) allowing residents to bring furniture and other personal items with them, (3) developing an informal atmosphere, and (4) providing individual rooms.

141. Tucker, N. J., and Smith, L. M. (1987). "All through the night." Geriatric Nursing, 8(5):256-257.

After several years of experiencing low morale and lack of cooperation with nursing assistants, the assistant director of nursing assessed the dismal work situation and recognized its underlying causes: rote care of residents irrespective of individual needs; poor structuring of routine assignments; and inefficient use of staff. The assistant director reported her observations and suggested a plan to change the situation. This change included more specific work routines and clearer time-lines to achieve these routines. Nursing assistants appreciated the fairness of the arrangement and the opportunities it gave them to relate to the residents.

142. Vivens, S., and Woolfork, C. (1983). "Nursing home admissions made more rational." Geriatric Nursing, 4(6):361-364.

To match applicants' needs with facility resources in advance, a refined admission process was developed including: preadmission home visit by a nurse and social worker, usually together; preadmission medical examination; admission conference among social worker and home visiting nurse and director of admissions; evaluation of the clinical load being carried by the home's various units; and involvement of the director of nursing, who decided on whether to accept or reject the applicant. Forms were developed to display and weigh the various pieces of information. This information provided the basis for the newly admitted resident's care.

143. Wagnild, G. (1988). "A descriptive study of nurse's aide turnover in long-term care facilities." Journal of Long-Term Care Administration, 16(1):19-23.

Reducing high turnover requires careful analysis of management practices, starting with recruitment and extending through orientation, staff development, supervision, employee compensation, and involvement of nurse's aides in management decisions.

144. Wallace, R. W., and Brubaker, T. H. (1984). "Long-term care with short term workers: An examination of nursing home nurse aide turnover." Journal of Applied Gerontology, 3(1):50-58.

Using secondary analysis of data generated from five nursing homes with common characteristics in a Midwestern state, this well-designed and carefully conducted study was undertaken to understand nursing assistant turnover. The sample consisted of 562 nursing assistants, 103 of whom were currently employed and 459 who had left their jobs. Most of the nursing assistants were under thirty years of age (55 percent), and had no dependent children (57 percent). The typical nursing assistant traveled six miles to work, had one year length of service at his or her previous job, and had three months employment tenure as a nursing assistant. Two significant findings were: the nursing assistants who had more dependent children, traveled shorter distances to work, and had a high number of months worked on a previous job tended to stay in the job longer; the older the nursing assistant the less likely the turnover; as the nursing assistant's employment tenure increased the decision to leave the job decreased; education was found not related to turnover. The authors suggest using these findings in recruiting nursing assistants and providing newly hired persons with clear definitions of their jobs, inservice training, and a sense of belonging.

145. Waxman, H. M., Carner, E. A., and Berkenstock, G. (1984). "Job turnover and satisfaction among nursing home aides." The Gerontologist, 24(5):503-509.

Interviews with 234 nursing assistants from seven Philadelphia-area randomly selected proprietary nursing homes revealed variability between nursing homes in job turnover rate, job satisfaction, and perception of themselves. Greater turnover occurred in better quality homes offering good wages and benefits.

A positive association found between turnover rates and the nursing assistants' perception of the homes' order, organization, and control indicates that job turnover would lessen if nursing assistants were more involved in the decision making. Instruments included a questionnaire on demographics, employment history, the Minnesota Satisfaction Scale, and the short form of the Moos Ward Atmosphere Scale.

146. Wolk, S., and Telleen, S. (1976). "Psychological and social correlates of life satisfaction as a function of residential constraint." Journal of Gerontology, 31(1):89-98.

This research sought to assess the level of life satisfaction and to determine the most important correlates of satisfaction in two environments. One environment had a clearly defined and enforced set of rules and the other environment did not. The findings suggested the higher constraining environment was associated with a lower level of satisfaction among the personnel.

147. Wright, L. K. (1988). "A reconceptualization of the 'negative staff attitudes and poor care in nursing homes' assumption." The Gerontologist, 28(6):813-820.

This article suggests that nursing home personnel, including nursing assistants, have had their attitudes about caring for the debilitated elderly measured inappropriately. The inappropriate measures have used negative stereotypes and inaccurate information about the aged. The author suggests that behavior be used instead of attitude, and the behavior required of staff to care for the residents successfully be specified. A comprehensive proposal for research is provided.

SUMMARY

The literature on the work environment of the nursing assistant depicted what this work environment actually is and suggested what it could become. The positive aspects of the actual environment included opportunities to do humanitarian work; to work as a health care team member; and to aspire for greater responsibility, recognition, and pay. The negative aspects of the environment pertained to the excessive demands this environment made of the nursing assistant.

The literature also pointed up concern about the work environment's ability to provide high-quality and effective care for residents, especially when high staff turnover and low morale are commonplace. Suggestions on improving the quality of care were made, and these improvements should positively influence the work environment of the nursing assistant.

III
Training the Nursing Assistant

Preservice and inservice training are necessary to enhance the practice of nursing assistants. They must acquire the knowledge and skill necessary not only to provide the physical care of residents but also to provide psychosocial care. Such training should:

- Orient and prepare newly hired nursing assistants to be competent, efficient, and effective.
- Provide technical growth and career development.
- Assure high standards of service delivery and performance.

BOOKS

148. Blau, D., and Freed, A. O. (editors) (1979). <u>Mental health in the nursing home: An educational approach for staff</u>. Brookline, Mass.: Boston Society for Gerontologic Psychiatry. 138 Pp.

This manual contains six papers authored by different mental health practitioners. The Boston Society for Gerontologic Psychiatry conducted a series of workshops on mental health for nursing home personnel over a period of several years. The papers of this volume were written for those workshops. A variety of teaching methods were used at the workshops along with the presentation and discussion of the papers. They included: role playing and the use of videotapes. The topics covered by the papers are: psychological problems of residents in their adjustment to the nursing home, the nursing home as a community, the resident as a person, the resident's family, the nursing home staff as a team, treatable dementias in the elderly, dying and death in a nursing home, and the work stresses of nursing home personnel.

149. Brody, E. M. (1977). <u>Long-term care of older people: A practical guide</u>. New York: Human Sciences Press. 402 Pp.

This book contains the historical background and development of long-term care facilities and their current goals and programs. Particular attention is given to the provision of social work services and to program development and operations. The book also has two guest chapters by Stanley J. Brody on resources for long-term care in the community and policy issues in long-term care.

150. Caldwell, E., and Hegner, B. R. (1969). <u>Health assistant</u>. Albany, N.Y.: Delmar Publishers. 221 Pp.

This text is intended to provide beginning nursing assistants with the initial skills and background information necessary to function as assistants to the professional nursing staff.

151. Cherescawich, G. D. (1964). <u>A textbook for nursing assistants</u>. St. Louis: C. V. Mosby. 468 Pp.

This text deals with the basic nursing responsibilities and techniques for the nursing assistant. Its major focus is on meeting the physical needs of residents; however, some attention is given to their emotional needs, and providing care for dying residents.

152. Conahan, J. M. (1976). <u>Helping your elderly patients: A guide for nursing assistants</u>. New York: Tiresias Press. 128 Pp.

This guide seeks to help nursing assistants understand their important role when caring for elderly persons, and to increase their sensitivity to the needs of elderly residents of nursing homes. Accordingly, the guide contains material on the needs of the elderly and ways of helping them. Emphasis is placed on communicating with them, and making diagnostic observations to use in caring ways. Role playing for inservice training is included as a means of helping nursing assistants learn how to handle real life situations in the living units for the elderly.

153. Cosella, C. (1979). <u>Training exercises to improve interpersonal relations in health organizations.</u> Greenvale, N.Y.: Panel Publishers. 404 Pp.

This manual contains thirty six exercises organized into eleven chapters for employees to improve their interpersonal relations in the workplace. Introductory written material, detailed instructions, and supporting forms to be completed by trainees (in class) are included. The topics of the chapters include: the individual and the group, the individual in organizations, interpersonal and organizational communication, leadership, conflict management, organizational climate, managing innovation and change, team building, and problems and problem solutions. An instructor's manual is available: Gilbert, J. G. (1977). <u>The Paraprofessional and the Elderly.</u> Greenvale, N.Y.: Panel Publishers.

154. Denham, M. J. (editor) (1983). <u>Care of the long-stay elderly patient.</u> London: Groom Helm (U.S. distributor Sheridan House), 145 Palisade St., Dobbs Ferry, N.Y.). 236 Pp.

This edited book contains thirteen chapters contributed by different authors and coauthors. The editor provides two chapters that give the book its framework and direction. Its concern is for a positive program for the acute medical and psychiatric problems of the elderly, particularly in Great Britain; however, its substance is relevant to nursing home care in the United States. Though the book's interest is practical--improving the patient's quality of life in long-stay care--it carefully refers to a substantial amount of U.S. as well as British research and practice literature. Two chapters --one reviews long-term care in Europe and one considers long-stay institutions in the United States--give the book a cross-national perspective.

155. Didactic Systems. (1988). <u>How to be a nurse's aide in a nursing home--Instructor's guide.</u> Washington, D.C.: American Health Care Association. 221 Pp.

This instructor's guide is designed to assist staff development coordinators in organizing, planning, and conducting a preservice training program using <u>How to be a nurse's aide in a nursing home</u> as a text, also published by the American Health Care Association.

156. Donovan, J. E., Belsjoe, E. H., and Dillon, D. (1978). The nurse assistant. Second edition. New York: McGraw-Hill. 404 Pp.

    This text is an introduction to work as a nursing assistant. Along with covering basic nursing procedures, it has chapters on caring for the geriatric resident and caring for the dying resident.

157. Ernst, N. S., and West, H. L. (1983). Nursing home staff development. New York: Springer. 132 Pp.

    This book provides an overview of the educational components involved in inservice training, its development, delivery, and evaluation. Particular attention is given to several teaching techniques; for example, lecture, role playing, case study, simulation, and drawing on resources outside the facility including community college courses and consultants.

158. Fasano, M. A. (1980). Nurse assistant in long term care: A workbook and instructional program. Second edition, Sacramento, Calif.: InterAge. 174 Pp.

    This is a textbook for nursing assistants. It outlines physical care measures and illustrates them.

159. Flack, M., and Johnston, M. (1986). Handbook for care: Practical guidelines for care assistants, nursing auxiliaries, and all assistants in health care. Beaconsfield, Bucks, England: Beaconsfield. 164 Pp.

    This handbook is designed to serve as a reference source for nursing assistants. It seeks to enhance the assistants' understanding of the residents' needs more fully and develop their skills in assisting the residents in residential care. After setting forth the role of the nursing assistant, it presents the importance of the nursing assistant's effectively communicating with others and cites techniques for doing so. Considerable attention is given to helping residents with their physical needs, providing a safe and therapeutic environment, and responding to the resident as a person with individual values and anxieties.

160. Flaherty, M. O. (1980). The care of the elderly person: A guide for the licensed practice nurse. Third edition. St. Louis: C. V. Mosby. 218 Pp.

This book was written to help practical nurses care for the elderly. Particular attention is given to the physical care of nursing home residents.

161. Gilbert, J. G., and Sullivan, C. M. (1976). The mental health aide. New York: Springer. 118 Pp.

This book was written especially for persons who are entering or planning to enter the mental health field as aides. It offers the new worker some understanding of a mental health center/hospital, the duties of a mental health aide, and some of the kinds of patients she is likely to encounter.

162. Hall, B. H., Gaingemi, M., Norris, V., Vail, V. H., and Sawatsky, G. (1952). Psychiatric aide education. New York: Grune and Stratton. 168 Pp.

This reports an experimental training program for psychiatric aides conducted by the Menninger Foundation in cooperation with the Topeka State Hospital. The historical background of the program is covered as are the recruitment and selection procedures, the program's curriculum including its clinical aspects, the techniques of teaching psychiatric aides, the promotion of learning through the program "structure," and the spirit of the program. Conclusions about the program are offered and recent developments in psychiatric aide education are discussed.

163. Houle, C. O. (1972). The design of education. San Francisco: Jossey-Bass. 323 Pp.

This book presents a model of adult education using the major decision points in planning and conducting a program. The items include: a possible educational activity is identified; a decision is made to proceed; objectives are identified and refined; a suitable format is designed that includes several elements (resources, leaders, methods, schedule, sequences, social reinforcement, individualization, roles and relations, criteria of evaluation, and clarity of design); the format is fitted into a larger pattern of life; the plan is put into effect; the results are measured and appraised; and the findings are fed back into the process as possible topics for further educational activity. The model is applied to several unique educational programs and to the major streams of thought

in adult education, including the work of such luminaries as John
Dewey, Kurt Lewin, Malcolm Knowles, and Kenneth Benne.

164. Huling, E. R. (1972). A manual of procedures for orderlies. St.
Louis: The Catholic Hospital Association. 105 Pp.

This manual is intended for training orderlies in hospitals.
Orderlies (nursing assistants) are seen as contributing to the
patients' quality of medical care. The manual has three parts: a
schedule of duties for orderlies, general nursing care procedures,
and special nursing procedures.

165. Hyman, R. T. (1970). Ways of teaching. Second edition.
Philadelphia: Lippincott. 371 Pp.

Now in its second edition, this book on educational methods
presents a conception of teaching that includes the elements of
the teacher, student, and subject matter. The teacher seeks to
convey knowledge, skills, and values primarily through language,
and involves the use of intelligence, reason, giving valid
information, and developing positive relations between the teacher
and student. Socratic dialogue, lecture, discovery, recitation,
sociodrama, and simulation are discussed in detail. In addition, the
book considers the "art of questioning" in the process of teaching.
Also, observing and evaluating teaching are presented.

166. Isler, C. (1973). The nurse aide. Second edition. New York:
Springer. 153 Pp.

In nineteen chapters, this book instructs the nursing assistant on
a broad range of activities; for example, her first day in the
hospital, becoming a part of the nursing staff, and a variety of
technical matters including the special needs of the elderly patient
and how to care for and help a dying patient.

167. Jodais, J. (1970). Personal care of patients: A text for health
assistants. Philadelphia: W. B. Saunders. 292 Pp.

This book was written to help nursing assistants understand the
principles of basic patient care. It also includes material on the
specific aspects of care: helping the patients with moving about,
caring for themselves, consuming food and fluids, and elimination
and toileting. Special chapters are offered on aging and on death.

168. Joyce, B., and Weil, M. (1986). Models of teaching. Third edition. Englewood Cliffs, N.J.: Prentice-Hall. 518 Pp.

This comprehensive treatment of the various approaches to teaching discusses their underlying theories, examines the research that has tested them, and illustrates how to use them. The approaches help students acquire information, ideas, skills, values, ways of thinking, and means of expressing themselves. The different approaches are cited for their advantages in achieving particular learning objectives; however, the reader is cautioned that no single model is the sole avenue to any given objective and that combinations of models are likely to have a more significant effect on learning than any one approach. The approaches of teaching are grouped into four "families" that categorize how people learn: the information processing family, the personal family, the social family, and the behavioral systems family.

169. Knoedler, E. L. (1958). The nursing assistant. Albany, N.Y.: Delmar. 101 Pp.

This manual focuses on training nursing assistants in the basic nursing skills and offers a number of units of instruction on elementary and more advanced nursing procedures.

170. Knowles, M. (1984). The adult learner: A neglected species. Third edition. Houston: Gulf. 292 Pp.

This book concentrates on developing an "andragogical model" of adult learning. It is presented as a "process" model in which the teacher (facilitator, consultant, charge agent) prepares in advance a set of procedures for involving the learners in a number of activities: (1) establishing a climate conducive to learning, (2) creating a mechanism for mutual planning, (3) diagnosing the needs for learning, (4) formulating program objectives that will satisfy these needs, (5) designing a pattern of learning experiences, (6) conducting these learning experiences with suitable techniques and materials, and (7) evaluating the learning outcomes and rediagnosing the learning needs. The andragogy model assumes students: (1) become increasingly self-directed, (2) are rich resources for learning, (3) profit from problem-centered teaching, (4) incorporate new social roles as a function of their learning, and (5) apply their learning immediately. Various learning theories are evaluated in the process of developing the andragogy theory of adult learning.

171. McClelland, L. H. (1971). Textbook for psychiatric technicians. C. V. Mosby. 269 Pp.

This is a comprehensive, easy-to-grasp text. It is divided into five parts: mental illness treated in the community and in the hospital, the role of the psychiatric technician, the therapeutic environment, understanding behavior, and patterns of behavior.

172. National Citizens' Coalition for Nursing Home Reform (NCCNHR). (1988). Final report, Nurse aide training symposium. Washington, D.C.: NCCNHR. 80 Pp.

Participants in the symposium explored a wide range of topics related to nurse aide training. The topics pointed directly at training included: What should the curriculum include? What should the qualifications of the teacher be? Where and when should the training be conducted? Should nurse aides be certified? How should training be tied to a career ladder? What is the cost of training and how best can it be met? Other related topics were considered: How can the poor image of nursing homes be improved? What kind of philosophy should the management have? What supports must the facility provide for the nurse aide? Should wages and benefits be raised? What is the practice scope of nurse aides? The major themes, including the agreements of the participants, are presented. Appendixes related to the content of the report and a selected bibliography are included. Also, an addendum on Public Law 100-203, Section 4211--Nursing Home Reform Act--follows the text of the report.

173. Reese, D. E. revised by Hughes, E., and Schrandt, J. (1988). How to be a nurse's aide in a nursing home--residential care procedures --student manual. Washington, D.C.: American Health Care Association. 117 Pp.

This manual was written to teach the essential skills needed by new nursing assistants working in resident care. Chapter topics include the nursing assistant's role, the resident's room, food and fluids, the resident's personal hygiene, bowel and bladder, positioning the patient, exercising the patient, control of disease and infection, the terminal patient, and fire safety.

174. Synder, R. E., and Ulmer, C. (1972). Guide to teaching techniques for adult classes. Englewood Cliffs, N.J.: Prentice-Hall. 64 Pp.

This is a brief practical guide for developing, carrying out, and evaluating classes for adults. The characteristics of learners, learning objectives, and techniques to implement programs are presented. Also, a teacher self-evaluation check list is provided.

175. Taber, M., et al. (1986). Handbook of practical care for the frail elderly. Phoenix, Ariz.: Oryx Press. 104 Pp.

This book was developed from a project to train nonprofessionals to assist elderly individuals who prefer to remain in their own homes. Sections cover basic tasks (meal planning, sanitation procedures) and physical conditions common among older people, and the psychosocial aspects of aging. Also, the interpersonal aspects of providing care to the frail elderly are covered.

176. Walsh, M. B., and Small, N. R. (editors) (1988). Teaching nursing homes: The nursing perspective. Owings Mills, Md.: National Health Publishing. 250 Pp.

This book incorporates material from eleven teaching nursing home sites and details the planning, implementing, administering, and evaluating of two specific sites: Georgetown University School of Nursing with the Greater Southeast Community Center for the Aging; and The Catholic University of America School of Nursing with the Carroll Manor Nursing Home. Overall, it provides a comprehensive analysis of the concept of a teaching nursing home.

177. Walston, B. J., and Walston, K. E. (1980). The nursing assistant in long-term care: A new era. St. Louis: C. V. Mosby. 204 Pp.

This is a self-help textbook for nursing assistants that describes the techniques and procedures involved in long-term care.

178. Weber, G. H., and McCall, G. J. (1987). The nursing assistant's casebook of elder care. Dover, Mass.: Auburn House. 227 Pp.

The book's focus is on the psychosocial aspects of nursing home care. Initial chapters present the nursing home as the context of the nursing assistant's work, residents' social and emotional needs and problems, role of the nursing assistant, ethical issues faced by the nursing assistant, and psychosocial techniques that the nursing assistant may use in helping the elderly. Also, material is presented on the use of the case study method as a procedure of teaching/learning. This material is followed by 105 cases drawn from two nursing homes by a research observer over a period of eight months. The cases are categorized in the areas of: (1) distressed feelings--loneliness, boredom, anxiety, anger and hostility, fear, unfounded bodily complaints, sadness, depression and suicide; (2) mental functioning--confusion/disorientation, self-doubt, excessive talking and justifying, overstriving to maintain independence, exaggerated claims about the virtues of others, avoidance and denial, displacement, suspicion and accusations, delusions and hallucinations; (3) stress between residents--argument, intimidation by attitude, physical threat, lack of interest, the put-down, constant hassle, breaking off, gossip, different resident psychologies; (4) stress between residents and nursing assistants --complaints about services and care, challenging the staff, blunders and abuse, complaints about the program, and excessive demands; (5) stress between resident and family--neglect, abandonment, possessions, demands, and uncertainty; (6) special care situations --belongings, resident noncompliance, sexual interest, selfish and self-indulgent residents, mismatch of home and resident, mentally ill residents, lack of cleanliness, incontinence, total care, and dying and death; and 7) things to feel good about--importance of work, friends among the staff, response by residents, administrative supports. The cases and questions following them are written to encourage the involvement and participation by nursing assistants in inservice training.

JOURNALS

179. Almquist, E., and Bates, D. (1980). "Training program for nursing assistants and LPNs in nursing homes." Journal of Gerontological Nursing, 6(10):622-627.

This report covers the experience of training programs to upgrade the skills of nursing paraprofessionals. It emphasizes the special problems of the geriatric patient. Conducted in Dade County, Florida, the training concentrated on four facilities within an eight-week period--six classes (one hour each session). All three shifts were included. The course syllabus covered two instructional units: the physiological background for the aging process; and the physical and psychosocial problems involved with aging, including their nursing implications. Three month followup surveys were requested of the directors of nursing and administrators of the facilities involved. A 50 percent response rate indicated that there were some improvements in job performance and positive changes in attitudes toward residents and other staff members.

180. Almquist, E., Stein, S., Weiner, A., and Linn, M. W. (1981). "Evaluation of continuing education for long-term care personnel: Impact upon attitudes and knowledge." Journal of the American Geriatric Society, 29(3):117-122.

Nursing assistants and licensed practical nurses (LPNs) from three proprietary nursing homes participated in a continuing education program designed to increase knowledge and enhance attitudes about the elderly in nursing homes. The program covered six weeks for the initial 115 nursing assistants and one full-day seminar for the 83 LPNs. The subject matter covered knowledge about human anatomy, the physiology of normal aging, physical and psychosocial problems of the elderly, and problems associated with cardiovascular accidents. The final participants, 29 nursing assistants and 52 LPNs, were tested before and after the training on their knowledge and attitudes toward the elderly. Results showed overall favorable changes for both nursing assistants and LPNs.

181. Barney, J. L. (1983). "A new perspective on nurse's aide training." Geriatric Nursing, 4(1):44-48.

The author argues that the training of nursing assistants must prepare them to serve as community surrogates in the places where the community's older citizens find themselves estranged, isolated, and powerless--nursing homes. In addition to knowledge and skills about resident care, the nursing assistant requires an equally important body of skills and knowledge about how to help the residents with their psychosocial needs.

182. Burke, R. E., D'Erasmo, M., and Burger, S. E. (1980). "Research brief: Training geriatric nursing assistants." Journal of Long-Term Care Administration, 8(3):37-40.

This article reports a pilot test of an inservice training program of geriatric nursing assistants. However, no data and very little qualitative information were reported. The curriculum emphasized: (1) the normal and abnormal aging processes influencing resident functional states; (2) a philosophy of care reflecting prevention of illness, improvement, and maintenance of resident functional states; and (3) nursing assistant intervention during encounters with residents to promote their wellness. Modules of curriculum were taught with: (1) minimal lecture and maximum student participation, (2) behavioral/action learner objectives and coordinated lesson plans, (3) flexible time requirements, and (4) continual reinforcement of previous learning. An unspecified evaluation system is recommended, but not reported on.

183. Buzzelli-Gibbons, K. (1981). "Formal training program for nurses aides." Nursing Homes, 30(5):2-3.

This article describes the planning, instruction, and evaluation by a director of inservice training of already employed and aspiring nursing assistants. These efforts reduced turnover and absenteeism, cut costs, and helped the trainees become more professional. The training was seventy-two hours extended over two months. The classes were limited to fifteen students. Even though the students paid for taking the course, they were not assured a job at the nursing home upon successfully completing the instruction. The curriculum included anatomy, physiology, the aging process, and the symptoms of diseases. Also, emphasis was placed on the emotional needs of residents and ways in which the nursing assistants could meet them. If trainees were hired, they were assigned to an experienced nursing assistant for up to four weeks, and evaluations by the director of inservice training were made until she considered the new employees fully competent to do the work. Qualitative observations of the nursing assistants' work by charge nurses and inspectors from the state health department have been highly favorable.

184. Campbell, M. E., and Browning, E. M. (1978). "Nursing assistants --An entrapped resource in providing quality care to the elderly ill." Journal of Gerontological Nursing, 4(6):18-20.

Based upon a workshop and related training experiences, the author recommended training in nursing homes for all levels of nursing personnel (including nursing assistants) to improve the quality of care provided the residents. The course work should emphasize positive aspects of aging, and the physical and psychological needs of the elderly. The training methods to achieve these objectives include lectures, films, demonstrations of physical and psychosocial techniques of nursing care, and group discussion on self-awareness. Such classroom substance and method should be augmented by highly skilled supervision on the job.

185. Catterson, J. (1983). "Nursing auxiliaries--Learning together." Nursing Times, 79(26):57-58.

The effort to train nursing auxiliaries (nursing assistants) by the East Leicestershire (England) Health District at local hospitals, rather than centrally at a particular location, began with a short trial course (content and length of time not given) in the autumn of 1978. After several intermediate steps to develop a comprehensive training program, the program consolidated its inservice training to reinforce the learning acquired during the auxiliaries' induction. It encourages the nursing auxiliaries to participate in their own training. This is in addition to lectures and clinical sessions on the wards. The participation technique asks the nursing auxiliaries to choose topics to think about and discuss at their next class session. The class sessions are held two hours a week for six weeks. The auxiliaries evaluated the course positively, though no data were given.

186. Cohen, M. D., Smyer, M. A., Garfein, A. J., Droogas, A., and Malone-Beach, E. E. (1987). "Perceptions of mental health training in nursing homes: Congruence among administrators and nurse's aides." Journal of Long-Term Care Administration, 15(2):20-25.

Questionnaires asked a sample of administrators and nursing assistants which of eleven disruptive mental health problems the nursing assistants were trained to manage. The problems were: threatening and abusive behavior, disoriented behavior, hallucinations and delusions, depression and withdrawal, suicidal behavior, agitation and wandering, problematic grief reactions, sensory deprivation, inappropriate sexual behavior, drug and alcohol abuse and misuse, and lack of family contact. Findings included: (1) the administrators and nursing assistants consistently disagreed on their perceptions of training received by the nursing assistants to deal with the eleven mental health problems--the administrators saw the nursing assistants' training to be adequate while the nursing assistants saw the training to be inadequate; (2) there was greater agreement among the nursing assistants in their responses than among the administrators on their perceptions of training received; and (3) there was considerable agreement between the two groups on the training methods used and the preferred training methods.

187. Crawford, S. A., Waxman, H. M., and Carner, E. A. (1983). "Using research to plan nurse aide training." American Health Care Association Journal, 9(1):59-61.

This article reports the experience of Thomas Jefferson University's Center for the Study of Geropsychiatry in developing a training program for nursing assistants. The authors took into account that nursing assistants make up only about 43 percent of all nursing home personnel yet deliver approximately 90 percent of the patient care; often are not trained to provide basic physical and psychosocial care; have a very high turnover rate; and are in need of esteem on the job. The authors also surveyed the nursing assistants about their job-related problems, and how they would organize the format and substance of training. Almost 80 percent indicated "working with difficult patients" as their highest problem. That was followed by "getting along with other aides," and "getting along with their supervisors." Details of the survey instrument were not provided, nor were other data analyses given. The authors' suggestions for training included: (1) combine didactic procedures that offer the "basics of care" with experimental ones to offer knowledge and skill about concrete work problems; (2) use teaching techniques appropriate for small groups and adaptable to situational changes; (3) provide curriculum materials about nursing home organization and its impact on the work of nursing assistants; and (4) increase the esteem of the nursing assistants.

188. Feldman, J., Burke, R., and Schwarzmann, J. (1978). "Analysis of training of unlicensed long-term-care personnel." Journal of Long-Term Care Administration, 6(2):1-12.

This research project sought to review all the published and unpublished preservice and inservice training materials of unlicensed long-term care workers. However, the lack of published material and unavailability of unpublished material reduced the intended scope of the review. Moreover, the review of collected material reflected entanglement, red tape, political and vested interests, and related problems associated with the management of training in long-term care.   A number of conclusions and recommendations were offered.

189. Goodwin, M., and Trocchio, J. (1987).   "Cultivating positive attitudes in nursing home staff."   Geriatric Nursing, 8(1):32-34.

A number of techniques are suggested to train nursing assistants to be positive in their work with residents: simulation games, inviting nursing assistants to act as residents for even a few hours but preferably for a few days; checklists for nursing assistants to review their skills; and group meetings for nursing assistants. The authors also indicated that professional nurses can promote positive attitudes by setting good examples, serving as exemplary role models, and demonstrating respect for one another and for nursing assistants.

190. Gutheil, I. A. (1985). "Sensitizing nursing home staff to residents' psychosocial needs." Clinical Social Work Journal, 13(4):356-367.

This is a case illustration in which a social work consultant provided inservice training to nursing assistants in a nursing facility to enhance their understanding of the residents in their care. Advantages of using inservice training are discussed, potential pitfalls are considered, and illustrations of training techniques are presented including dialoguing with nursing assistants, role playing, and helping nursing assistants listen to and communicate with residents.

191. Hameister, D. R. (1977).   "A design of inservice education for nurse's aides in a nursing home setting." Journal of Continuing Education in Nursing, 8(2):6-12.

This research clustered the tasks associated with the work of nursing assistants and considered their appropriateness for inclusion in an inservice training program. The clustering followed an analysis of questionnaire data gathered from 107 charge nurses and administrators chosen randomly from the nursing care facilities in Michigan. The highest ranking clusters included: personal hygiene; observation; analysis and interpretation; patient need for movement; nutrition and elimination; religious and spiritual needs; diagnostic activity; application of heat; cold and medical therapies; and oral and written communications. Considerations for making decisions about the content of specific nursing assistant training were discussed.

192. Headricks, M. M. (1982). "Determining the learning needs of nursing personnel in nursing homes." The Journal of Continuing Education in Nursing, 13(2):18-22.

The purpose of this study was to develop a means of identifying the learning needs of various groups of nursing personnel in nursing homes. Two assessment tools were used: Monette's self-fulfillment model (1977), in which the intent is to discover the felt needs of workers; and a nominal technique based upon a group process model for problem or need identification (Delbecq and Van de Van, 1971). Using these techniques with twelve RNs, ten LPNs, and forty NAs, the learning needs of each category of employees were identified. The nursing assistants indicated their greatest needs were to learn about the personal (mental stimulation, social interaction, leisure-recreational activity) and clinical physical needs of the elderly. Also, the nursing assistants expressed a need to learn about the residents' sensory and perceptive impairments.

193. Hickey, T. (1974). "In-service training in gerontology: Toward the design of an effective educational process." The Gerontologist, 5(2):57-64.

This article reports the first phase of a continuing education program for the providers of services to the elderly. The various issues of the undertaking are set forth, including: articulation of measurable goals for the several types of occupations included, routinizing the curriculum to provide a uniformly high quality of offerings to the enrollees, and the methodological problems of evaluation.

194. Hyerstay, B. J. (1978). "Political and economic implications of training nursing home aides." Journal of Nursing Administration, 8(6):22-24.

To provide training in the physical, social, and psychological aspects of care for nursing assistants would threaten the present nursing home industry. The increased knowledge and skill would disrupt the hierarchical arrangement of occupations and professions in the nursing home social structure. Increased wages would threaten the financial stability of the nursing home, overtax the meager resources of most residents, and make exceptional demands on the government for support. These changes would impact on the current political arrangements.

195. Jensen, D. L. (1977). "A continuing education opportunity for nursing assistants." Journal of Continuing Education in Nursing, 8(5):12-14.

The planning and implementation of a two-day workshop for nursing assistants on the etiology, symptomatology, and various therapies used with stroke victims are presented. An evaluation of the workshop was conducted. A second workshop was conducted on the care of the diabetic patient. Both workshops relied heavily on speakers with expertise in their respective topics.

196. Johnson, M. (1987). "A helping handbook." Senior Nurse, 6(2):11-12.

The author presents the major themes of the Handbook for Care (Beaconsfield, Bucks, England: Beaconsfield, 1986) written for auxiliaries (nursing assistants). Included in the contents are: roles for nursing auxiliaries, how to start training programs for nursing auxiliaries, what substance should be included in the programs, role of teachers, and performance review of the nursing auxiliaries' work.

197. Johnson-Pawlson, J., and Goodwin, M. (1986). "Total approach to nurse aide training." Provider, 12(8):16-18.

This article describes How to Be a Nurse Aide in a Nursing Home (student and instructor manuals), published by the American Health Care Association, and indicates that comprehensive training can make the difference between a quality nursing home and one that is substandard.

198. Korber, E. J. (1983). "Task analysis: Helping staff develop client independence." Nursing Homes, 32(2):32-34.

Training procedures are provided nursing assistants to teach elderly persons with organic syndromes such as Alzheimer's disease to feed themselves.

199. Linderman, H. (1985). "Training makes nursing assistants front line professionals." American Health Care Association Journal, 11(7):65-66.

This article reports on a program that combined inservice training and career ladder opportunities for nursing assistants, and suggests positive results.

200. Narayanasamy, S. A. (1985). "Evaluation of a training curriculum for nursing assistants." Nurse Education Today, 5(3):124-129.

This research suggests that a nursing assistant training program in Great Britain to care for mental patients was effective due to its teaching methods and curriculum content. Twenty-four nursing assistants were included in the study. A Likert-type scaled questionnaire was given to the nursing assistant after they completed their training.

201. Pembrey, S. (1986). "Project 2000: Who's helping whom?" Nursing Times, 82(38):48-49.

Given the various levels of knowledge, skills, decisions, and actions required in nursing care, the argument of the article is that patients' assistants (nursing assistants) with the right level of training, support, and supervision from professional nurses can carry out delegated tasks. Yet this article reflects doubt on whether nurses actually need nursing assistants.

202. Payne, M. B., and Lyons, J. D. (1987). "Preparation of geriatric aides for patient care and certification." Geriatric Nursing, 8(3):125-127.

This article describes the background and current status of a program to prepare nursing assistants for certification in New York State. Currently, the course is divided into two semesters with thirty semester hours making up each part. Part I deals with the role of the geriatric aide, the aging process, and the community and institutional environments. Part II focuses on health problems commonly seen in the elderly and specific nursing aide care techniques. Student learning is evaluated through written quizzes and a final examination. Also, students keep logs of their weekly homework assignments. The program has improved the nursing assistants' job satisfaction; however, it has not improved the turnover rate.

203. Rantz, M., and Roethle, L. (1984). "Who is my attendant today?" Geriatric Nursing, 5(3):187-189.

A pilot program was designed to determine whether a combination of written and verbal introductions of nursing assistants to residents would be more effective than a verbal introduction alone, as had been the practice in the past. The pilot test included two living units. One had plastic-covered cards taped to each resident's door at wheelchair or eye level, reading "I am your attendant," and the attendant's name. In addition, the nursing assistants introduced themselves to residents at the beginning of each shift. "My name is on your card so that any time you want to know who is helping you, look here." In the other unit, a verbal statement indicating who would be caring for each resident was given at the beginning of each shift and verbally reinforced throughout the shift. After two weeks it was determined that of the residents who were given written and verbal instructions, 42 percent were able to name or describe their nursing assistant for the shift. Of the residents who were given the name of their nursing assistant and had it repeated during the shift, only 27 percent of the responses were correct. Given these pilot test findings, the facility extended the use of written and verbal reinforcement throughout all living units. After twenty-four months, ninety-five residents were randomly selected and interviewed and a questionnaire was distributed to all employees for their reactions. Only 26 percent of the residents could correctly name or describe the employee caring for them that day, and 50 percent gave an incorrect answer; 23 percent could not communicate any response. One possible explanation is that the staff began to rely on the written instruction of the nursing assistant's identity and neglected verbal reinforcement.

204. Schwartz, A. N. (1974). "Staff development and morale building in nursing homes." The Gerontologist, 14(1):50-53.

This essay urges staff development by committed, articulate, on-site leaders who convey the home's mission as a daily reality by their own activity and dedication and by their encouragement, support, recognition, appreciation, and training of staff. The aim of staff development is to improve patient care and staff morale and to reduce turnover.

205. Skinkle, R. R., and Grant, P. R. (1988). "An outcome evaluation of an in-service training program for nursing home aides." Canadian Journal on Aging, 7(1):48-57.

Nursing home assistants are the primary care providers for the institutionalized elderly, but until recently, nursing assistants have received very little formal training. Recognizing this, some community colleges have implemented inservice training programs. This article presents the results of an impact assessment of a Saskatchewan program. Results indicated that program graduates knew significantly more about simple nursing skills, the aging process, and the philosophy of long-term care in comparison to nursing assistants from nursing homes that did not offer this inservice training.

206. Stein, K. Z. (1986). "Nursing assistants learn through the competency based approach." Geriatric Nursing, 7(4):197-200.

This article defines competency-based preemployment training and describes how one program used this approach to teach psychosocial skills to nursing assistant trainees in a long-term care facility. Trainees were enrolled in the program for four weeks. The program included forty hours of classroom instruction and 100 hours of clinical training under the supervision of a registered nurse. Trainees' written course evaluations, completed at the end of four weeks, showed that most felt the sequencing of training helped them apply their knowledge to the clinical setting and understand the elderly persons' needs. At the end of the training, most trainees were hired for the evening or night shift.

207. Wallace, C. (1984). "Sicker patients spur teaching links." Modern Healthcare, 14(7):58.

This article argues that nursing homes will be caring for sicker patients as hospitals discharge them sooner to get the hospital costs below the fixed reimbursement rates of Medicare's prospective payment system. Further, it argues that the demand of caring for sicker patients will encourage more nursing homes to affiliate with medical and nursing schools to increase their staffs and overall skills to care for the sicker patients. Further, the nursing homes would provide the medical and nursing schools on-site training for their students and a place to conduct research on long-term care.

208. Woolfork, C. H. (1988). "An in-service program that worked." Geriatric Nursing, 9(2):94-97.

This essay urges inservice education to present both required information (federal regulation on staff development--CFR 405.1121[h]) and related information in a manner to promote attendance, encourage participation, and improve the quality of patient care. In-home and community resources are seen as cost-effective. Particular attention is given to mental health principles to conduct rap and support groups for nursing assistants and RNs.

SUMMARY

Training the nursing assistant in basic nursing care and psychosocial skills was covered by the literature. This need was cited frequently and various preservice and inservice training projects were described. A number of training techniques--lecture, discussion, demonstrations, role playing, supervised practice, individual reading, and so on--were considered for their most appropriate use.

Many programs were organized experientially and reported by essay. They were primarily qualitative. Only occasionally were projects organized experimentally and analyzed statistically.

IV
Advocacy and Bargaining

Nursing assistants must speak out to improve their working conditions, salaries, and benefits, and to enhance the care of the elderly, and have others do so. Though sometimes difficult, in the case of the nursing assistants it is necessary. Advocacy and bargaining are particular ways of speaking out. Advocacy refers to expressing a view, urging an action or several actions. Here it concerns the nursing assistants' saying that their psychosocial practice, working conditions, and pay are in need of improvement and that the steps necessary to enhance them should be taken. Bargaining concerns the negotiations between the nursing assistants, or someone representing them, and the nursing home administration and owner to effect improvements of the type mentioned.

BOOKS

209. Bacharach, S. B., and Lawler, E. J. (1981). <u>Bargaining: Power, tactics, and outcomes</u>. San Francisco: Jossey-Bass. 234 Pp.

This book presents bargaining as the interplay between parties in which each analyzes his or her bargaining power in relation to the bargaining power of the opponent. The book's framework suggests that dependence (parties having a stake in the bargaining relationship) underlies bargaining and drives the tactical and subjective nature of bargaining. A number of additional topics are considered, for example, procedures of argument, techniques of conflict resolution, and the dynamics of making concessions.

210. Druckman, D. (editor) (1977). <u>Negotiations: Social-psychological perspectives</u>. Beverly Hills, Calif.: Sage. 416 Pp.

This book of thirteen chapters by various experts and a comprehensive introduction and a conclusion by the editor provides a thorough coverage of its topic. Subjects of concern on negotiations include: objectives, incentives, and conflict; processes, strategies, and outcomes; influences, conditions, and background factors; and complex settings and processes. The text is clear, well organized, and well documented.

211. Ilich, J. (1973). <u>The art and skill of successful negotiation</u>. Englewood Cliffs, N.J.: Prentice-Hall. 205 Pp.

In fifty two short chapters this book discusses such questions as deciding the time and place to negotiate, whether or not to have the client present, how to develop a good negotiating memory, how to select technical assistance for the negotiation, how to develop a negotiation strategy, how to determine the final negotiating authority, how to dispose of potentially troublesome arguments, how to handle anger in negotiation, and other situational factors involved in negotiation.

212. Metzger, N., and Pointer, D. D. (1985). <u>Labor relations and personnel management in long-term health care facilities</u>. Washington, D.C.: American Health Care Associations. 128 Pp.

This book provides the administrator with information about administrative procedures and legal requirements of dealing with labor unions. Chapters include preventive labor relations, personnel administration, grievance procedures, union organizing strategy and tactics, structure and functions of the nation's labor law, collective bargaining, unfair labor practices, labor management disputes, provisions of the labor-management reporting and disclosure act, negotiating, and living with the collective bargaining agreement.

213. Strauss, A. (1979). <u>Negotiations: Varieties, contexts, processes, and social order</u>. San Francisco: Jossey-Bass. 275 Pp.

The suggested framework of negotiation is broad. It takes into account negotiation settings, objectives being sought, and several types of negotiations (appeal to authority, coercion, and force).

The author's framework is used to analyze pertinent research literature and analyze instances of negotiation that have occurred in politics, industry, and international affairs.

214. Walster, E., Walster, G. W., and Berscheid, E. (1978). Equity: Theory and research. Boston, Mass.: Allyn and Bacon. 312 Pp.

This volume presents the theory of equity and the research that has been conducted to describe its application and test its validity.

215. Weber, G. H., and McCall, G. J. (editors) (1978). Social scientists as advocates: Views from the applied disciplines. Beverly Hills, Calif.: Sage. 215 Pp.

This is a collection of original articles on advocacy designed to indicate the conceptions, strategies, and tactics of the several social sciences. Intended as a resource for educators and practitioners, it presents the views of applied anthropology, community psychology, law, social work, applied sociology, and urban planning.

216. Young, O. R. (editor) (1975). Bargaining: Formal theories of negotiations. Urbana, Ill.: University of Illinois Press. 412 Pp.

With an introduction and conclusion by the editor, this volume includes eighteen authored and coauthored articles (two of which have comment or rejoinders) written mainly by economists. Though recognition is given to less formal analyses of bargaining than "deductive models," the substance of the book tilts very much in that direction. A general familiarity with the principal techniques used in game-theoretic and economic models will prove helpful to the reader.

JOURNALS

217. Berger, S G. (1987). "How nurses relate to nursing assistants." Provider, 13(4):14-17.

The nurse's responsibility to the nursing assistant is considered in regard to recruitment, orientation, establishment of a positive working environment, training, supervision, and evaluation. The establishment of a positive environment includes the director of nursing serving as an advocate for the nursing assistant in two broad areas: resident advocacy and staff advocacy. Resident advocacy pertains to such matters as ensuring the availability of supplies and equipment and sufficient numbers of nursing staff with appropriate skills to meet residents' needs. Staff advocacy includes pressing for a nursing assistant promotional-career ladder with commensurate pay increases and benefits, and if such is established, maintaining it. Also, the director of nurses must empower the nursing assistants to report their observations at staff meetings and case conferences, and in shift reports.

218. Butler, R. N. (1980). "The alliance of advocacy with science." The Gerontologist, 20(2):154-162.

This article casts the current relationship between advocacy and science into its historical context and illustrates the positive consequences of the alliance between advocacy and science, particularly the national programs for the elderly.

219. Efthim, A. (1968). "The nonprofessionals revolt." The Nation, 207(3):70-72.

This article reports the advocacy and bargaining efforts of the nonprofessionals (mainly nursing assistants) at the Topeka State Hospital to improve the patients' care and the nursing assistants' working conditions and career prospects. Techniques used by the nonprofessionals were confrontation, use of the press and the generation of public opinion, a strike, and negotiation.

220. Evans, L. K. (1986). "Beyond tradition into the future." Provider, 12(8):4-6.

This is the introductory article to the issue, "Long Term Care Nursing Comes of Age." The author explains that traditional roles of the caregivers are too limited. In addition to having the caregivers generate more sophisticated conceptions of care, including psychosocial care, he argues for them to develop greater leadership and management skills through education and training.

221. Kassoris, M. D. (1967). "The San Francisco Bay area 1966 nurses." Monthly Labor Review, 90(6):8-12.

Though concerned with nurses, this case study has relevance for the issues and concerns of nursing assistants. It focuses on ward discontent by nurses, the evolution of bargaining, the work of a fact-finding panel, and the consequences of its findings.

222.   Kheel, T. W., and Kaden, L.B. (1970). "A plan to resolve impasses in hospital bargaining." Labor Monthly Review, 93(4):45-48.

This article proposes creating a board to promote collective bargaining in hospitals and health services with the primary function of prompting joint decisionmaking by mutual agreement of the workers and management. This board would be designated as the agent to decide when direct negotiations are no longer possible or productive and to determine what procedure should be followed as an alternative. Further, the board should be able to restrain a strike for a limited amount of time, perhaps twenty days, to give it time to consider the next steps that might be taken. Finally, the board would have power to submit any remaining issues to arbitration.

223.   Tully, C. T. (1985). "A proposal for a nonreinstatement rule in unfair labor practice cases involving patient abuse." American Journal of Law and Medicine, 11(3):319-341.

In 1974 Congress passed the Health Care Institutions Amendments, which granted to nonprofit health care workers collective organizing and bargaining rights very similar to those that workers in other industries have enjoyed for decades under the National Labor Relations Act. Congress intended to give health care workers only that degree of parity compatible with the provision of high-quality patient care. For example, Congress required health care workers to provide ten days advance notice of an intent to strike to ensure that the continuity of patient care would not be disrupted. The agency charged with enforcing the act, the National Labor Relations Board, has failed to distinguish employee misconduct in industrial settings from patient abuse in health care because of union activities. The board has typically ordered the reinstatement of nonguilty workers, with back pay. The author of the article suggests that a front-pay remedy is more appropriate to these cases because it protects the patient's right to be free from abuse without sacrificing employee unionization rights.

SUMMARY

The literature on advocacy and bargaining suggests that they are underdeveloped and underused procedures for nusing assistants, but their potential is clear given their successful use by other occupations.

V
Toward a Psychosocial
Model of Practice

A model of practice is a prototype, a conceptual construction that brings together the most promising services of an occupation or profession to help its clients. It stems from practice experience, research, theory, and ideology and values. Further, not only must the model pull its various parts together into a congruent whole, but it must also fit itself into the parent organization, especially the organization's objectives and division of work.

VALUES AND IDEOLOGY

The values of nursing assistant practice include benevolence, compassion, and respect for the elderly, especially the frail, ill, and dependent who should be cared for with regard and intelligence. Moreover, care should include the elderlys' physical as well as psychosocial needs to enhance their quality of life, improve or stabilize their condition, or ease their dying. As members of the nursing home health care team, the nursing assistants working with the nurses, physicians, adjunctive therapists, and administrators believe in service, cooperation, and participating in the decisions regarding the residents' care. These values and beliefs support diligent, responsible, and competent work, and in addition, inspiration and perseverance.

PERTINENT RESEARCH FINDINGS

The special importance of the nursing assistants to residents is generally acknowledged (Institute of Medicine, 1986; National Citizens'

Coalition for Nursing Home Reform, 1988). Yet Klus and Thoreson (1980) document the nursing assistant's life of uncertainty marked by grievance, absenteeism, and turnover. Others (Institute of Medicine, 1986; Gale, 1973) cite exceptionally heavy work demands, lack of regard, and low pay. Brannon, et al. (1988) indicate the need for redesigning the job of the nursing assistant. LeSar (1987) urges developing the nursing assistant job as a creditable and rewarding career. Training and improving working conditions and pay are common recommendations. Bye and Iannone (1987) in judging the excellence of nursing assistant care use the criteria of nursing assistants' conveying a caring attitude and consistently giving safe, efficient, and effective care. Fisk (1984) also recommends a caring attitude. Wagnild and Manning (1986) reaffirm conveying respect to the residents. Almquist and Bates (1980) consider the attitudes of the nursing assistant toward the residents, as well as their knowledge of the aging process and basic nursing skills, as important. Weber and McCall (1987) emphasize the psychosocial aspects of the nursing assistants' work. Dawes (1981) urges including the nursing assistants in the nursing home health care team, typically made up of the physicians, nurses, and adjunctive therapists. Handschu (1973) suggests expanding the role of the nursing assistant to the role of psychosocial companion to the residents. Several researchers would equip the nursing assistants with behavioral management skills (Mueller and Atlas, 1972; Rinke, Williams, Lloyd and Smith-Scott, 1978; Sand and Berni, 1974; and Schnelle and Traughber, 1983). Blau and Freed (1979) recommend that nursing assistants use mental health methods in their work.

THE NURSING HOME OBJECTIVES AND DIVISION OF WORK

The nursing home must provide rehabilitation to those elderly who can respond, care and comfort to those whose health can be maintained, and comfort to those who are dying. Basic nursing care, headed by nurses and assisted by nursing assistants and adjunctive therapists, and the overall direction of physicians, are the regimen of service. The nursing assistant assists the nurse, and in so doing she plays a number of roles.

The nursing home must: invite the nursing assistants to participate in developing the residents' care plans including setting realistic but high objectives of care; encourage the nursing assistants to interact openly and extensively with the home's nurses to effect the objectives of care; require progressively greater skill from nursing assistants and couple that with a career ladder; press the nursing assistants for responsible self-monitoring of their work performance; encourage confidence and trust between superiors and subordinates; and provide nursing assistants a reasonable work load and adequate pay.

The Helping Roles of the Nursing Assistant

Drawing from role theory (Biddle, and Thomas, 1966), the nursing assistant may be viewed as playing a number of roles in her job. She is an assistant, a cleaner and custodian, an attendant, a diagnostician decision maker, a deliverer of physical care, a communicator and counselor. These roles are typically entertwined in the nursing assistant's daily work. More specifically, the roles engage a number of activities.

As an assistant the nursing assistant helps the charge nurse carry out the nursing care responsibilities of the living unit or ward. This is a broad role as it requires such simple skills as resident bathing and cleaning, and complex skills such as catheter care and assisting those residents receiving oxygen. This role may also be viewed as a deliverer of physical care.

Cleaner and Custodian roles engage the nursing assistant in janitorial duties, particularly if the nursing home does not employ orderlies to do such work. These roles require cleaning the residents' rooms, toilets, showers, and baths. Custodial duties include maintaining a safe and secure physical environment. Fire safety and disaster assistance must be practiced.

The attendant role overlaps the role of assistant because it refers to the nursing assistants' attending to the residents in the activities of basic nursing care--serving, being present, and so on.

Diagnostician decision maker role asks the nursing assistant to contribute to the residents' plan of care. Observations of residents' ambulation, dexterity, mood, mental response, interest, relationships, and general health are necessary for planning and providing daily care. The nursing assistants' first-hand and continuous contact with the residents gives them an excellent opportunity to observe the residents' characteristics and care needs.

Cutting across all of the nursing assistants' duties is decision making, including: What to conclude about a resident's behavior, determining the effectiveness of psychosocial approaches in working with a resident, how to apply a technique suggested by the charge nurse, and how to interpret the report of a fellow nursing assistant about her observations of a resident. Moreover, she must find ways to help when residents refuse to get up, become incontinent, cannot find the dining room, cannot sleep, grieve over their families' failure to visit, argue with other residents, make excessive demands for personal care, imagine illnesses and demons, and fear death.

The communicator role engages the nursing assistant with other staff, occasionally someone in the administrative hierarchy, residents, and sometimes with members of the resident's family. The role demands being a careful listener--one who is sensitive to what is being said and what is not being said (which may be exceedingly important); and a careful talker--one who is spontaneous yet reflective in what she says. Such communication carries attitudes and feelings, so important in talking with residents who need their spirits lifted, fears reduced, anxieties quieted, suspicions allayed, and courage bolstered.

The counselor role is broad in scope and pertains especially to the residents' psychosocial needs. It encompasses aspects of several other roles, especially diagnostician, decision maker, and attendant. The diagnostic role would be used to assess the resident's emotional state; manner of thinking; interpersonal relations with other residents, staff, and family.

In role of a counselor, the nursing assistant engages the residents psychosocially in a number of helpful ways including being empathic, serving as a stable model, and responding with tact.

The nursing assistant may respond to the different residents in a variety of ways. To the confused resident she may clarify muddled situations and affirm the resident's efforts. Self-doubting and very uncertain residents may be helped by psychosocial support and encouragement. The defensiveness of overly talkative and self-justifying residents may be reduced by the nursing assistant's listening matter of factly. If a resident avoids and denies the significance of any matter that arouses anxiety, the nursing assistant may gently help her face the matter. Residents who push their basic problems onto the immediate situation may respond positively to a friendly query from the nursing assistant about the matter of concern, and to help from the nursing assistant to explore it. The suspicious resident and the complexities of the behavior suggest a cautious, matter-of-fact approach by the nursing assistant. Reassurance may be helpful to the resident but the nursing assistant must exercise care not to become ensnarled in the resident's preoccupation.

The nursing assistant will encounter residents who argue with each other. She might hear them out, respond to objective aspects of their arguments, and disregard the other matters. If they threaten each other physically, the nursing assistant must intervene, stop the threat, and then, with the assistance of the charge nurse, work out the issues.

The residents may lack an interest in relating to and interacting with others. They should be introduced to others and encouraged to extend themselves and engage in activities, especially those that involve others.

Some residents may put others down. The nursing assistant must tactfully call it to their attention and help them develop other ways of relating to others. Or they may constantly argue and hassle each other. They may be permitted to continue if they seem to get satisfaction out of their exchanges. However, if the hassling is demeaning, one-sided, or harsh, the residents should be encouraged to settle their argument (if such is possible). If the residents continue they should be encouraged to pursue separate activities.

A few residents will hurt others with gossip. They should be discouraged from generating and passing gossip, and be involved in constructive activity. Gossip and rumors are part of group life. The nursing assistant must be careful not to overreact, but if residents are being embarrassed or hurt, she should talk with the persons involved.

Some residents have very different psychological makeups and do not get along with each other. The nursing assistant should encourage the residents to work out their differences and conduct their relationships on matters of general agreement. If such is not possible, separate activities for each may be the preferred action, or assignment to different rooms if they are roommates.

Complaints about the service and care may be voiced by the residents. The nursing assistant must hear them out in order to understand the dissatisfaction fully and give the residents an opportunity to ventilate their feelings. Further, the nursing assistant must guard against being defensive or angered by such complaints. Instead, she needs to give the complaints serious consideration, make corrections if she can, perhaps discuss them with the charge nurse to get some counsel and assistance, and with other nursing assistants for ideas and support. Moreover, if the changes desired by the resident cannot be made, she should advise the resident. If the residents' complaints are chronic and unfounded, the nursing assistant may choose not to respond with the assumption that the lack of response will discourage the complaining, or she may advise the residents that their constant complaining is not appropriate. There are occasions when a complaint is symbolic of something else; that is, the subject of the complaint is not the real subject of the resident's dissatisfaction. On such occasions the resident might be referred to the social worker.

The resident's challenge to the nursing assistant's authority and/or credibility must be met tactfully by the nursing assistant to preserve her stature and effectiveness. As difficult as it may be, the nursing assistant should feel secure in the face of the resident's challenge, and must be careful not to overreact with anger, threats, or rejection. Specifically, the nursing assistant must carefully evaluate and clarify the challenge with the resident, make amends (if such are indicated), suggest the resident make amends (if such are indicated and the resident does not volunteer to make them), and carry on with dignity and confidence.

A resident's excessive demands may stem from pain or anxiety, or from a character-conditioned way of getting her way. Intense or aggravating pain requires additional care or medical attention. Anxiety may be alleviated by reassurance. An unrealistic character-conditioned demand might be ignored.

The counselor role also requires the nursing assistant to confront herself on such matters as blunders and abuse. Recognizing and admitting either a blunder or abuse is difficult even to one's self, yet admitting such to herself and the charge nurse, making amends, committing herself to an improved practice, and seeking the necessary skills is the way to proceed. Of the two behaviors, blunders are usually easier to cope with because they imply no malice. They are "goofs" that typically cause little damage and can be corrected easily. Abuse is intentionally harming a resident, vindictively. That is a serious matter. The abuse must be talked through with the charge nurse. The director of nursing and the nursing home's administrator will also become involved. The details of the abuse, and questions of retaining or discharging the nursing assistant, making amends, and preventing future abuse must be considered in detail.

The counselor role, on occasion, will involve the family of the resident, even though this task is assigned to either the charge nurse or the social worker. As the nursing assistant may be in the living unit during family visits, this makes her a likely person for the family to ask about the resident's welfare, the administration of the nursing home, and the program. Except on routine matters of care, the nursing assistant should refer questions to the charge nurse.

CAREER OPPORTUNITIES TO SUPPORT THE MODEL OF PRACTICE

A nursing assistant career--that is, a nursing assistant's being able to work in the occupation over a period of years with increasing proficiency, responsibility, pay, and esteem depends--on the policies of the nursing home. Specifically, the nursing home must provide a reasonable and varied work schedule to challenge the nursing assistant, and encouragement and support. Such provisions include pre- and inservice training, consultation and supervision, adequate pay and recognition, and opportunities to advance. Given the inadequacy of regulations that govern nursing homes, and the lack of a broad union base or trade association representation, a great deal of the responsibility for developing the nursing assistants' career opportunities rests with the administration of nursing homes.

KNOWLEDGE AND SKILL DEVELOPMENT

The nursing assistants' knowledge and skill are mainly derivatives from the professional armamentarium of nursing. However, the undeveloped character of the nursing assistant occupation has drawn only modestly from human anatomy and physiology, personality theory, and knowledge about the impact of aging and disease. Similarly, the nursing assistant usually shares only a limited number of skills taken from the nurses' battery of patient care skills.

Academically, the prospects of using derivative knowledge from nursing are substantial, especially if there are auspices to encourage it and the professional motivation to accomplish it. The major challenge lies in developing the psychosocial details of the nursing assistant's work, particularly the generation and maintenance of a therapeutic milieu. Among the necessary items to be developed are devising a conceptual scheme to designate types of situations and behavior that call for specific actions by the nursing assistant to achieve particular ends. This concept implies original work and research to test its quality.

SUMMARY

A concept of nursing assistant psychosocial practice was presented. Elements considered included values and ideology, pertinent research findings, nursing home objectives and division of work, helping roles, career opportunities to support the model of practice, and knowledge and skill development.

VI
Models to Enhance Practice

This chapter presents several ways to improve the practice of nursing assistants. Inservice training is suggested as one way, and it may take many different approaches. Only two are considered here; one uses a human relations method of teaching and the other uses a behavioral method. Both approaches aim to achieve the same objectives and use the same curriculum materials.

Another possible way to improve the practice of nursing assistants is through developing the overall organization of the nursing home and giving particular attention to the work of the nursing assistants. Like the variety of ways to conduct inservice training, there are a variety of ways to organize and carry out an organizational development plan. Two approaches will be presented: one in which the development plan is organized and conducted in-house, under the leadership of a nursing home staff member; and another in which an outside consultant leads the planning and implementation of the plan under an agreement with the nursing home. Both approaches are focused on the same objectives and use essentially the same procedures.

The third and fourth ways to improve the practice of nursing assistants are by advocacy and bargaining. Advocacy is proposed for application to two different settings; one in which the advocacy is a legitimate way of proceeding, and the other in which advocacy is not legitimate. On bargaining a particular approach is suggested--a rational equity model.

Before these several ways to improve the practice of nursing assistants are presented, factors to consider in developing an approach for use in a specific nursing home are set forth.

FACTORS TO CONSIDER IN DEVELOPING A MODEL

A State of Awareness and Tension as Prerequisites

Disparity between what is and what ought to be must enter the consciousness of one or more persons to cause tension and initial action. Initially, the concern is likely to be discussed with others who are in a position to observe and perhaps experience the phenomena of concern. The concern might be the nursing assistants' poor psychosocial skills in working with the residents, or the nursing home's failure to include the nursing assistants in planning the residents' care, or the nursing assistants' poor pay. The shared concern must be articulated so it can be tackled. Without such spelling-out and accompanying tension, nothing is likely to happen. Even with them, gaining a state of awareness is the first of many steps in constructing and implementing an intervention.

Definition of the Problem

Though the problem of nursing assistants may be clearly apparent--inadequate training, poor wages, poor working conditions, the lack of respect by the professionals, or the absence of career mobility--it requires: detailing, especially as it exists in a nursing home. Also involved is a preliminary consideration of what might be done to solve the problem.

Deliberations Involve Values

Values--the worthwhileness of a problem and of various possible solutions--are inexorably entwined in planning an intervention. Concerned about implicit in contrast to explicit values, Myrdal (1944) urged that persons pursuing social problems make their value premises explicit so that they and others know the most powerful influences on decisionmaking. Such explicitness can help the developers of interventions discover their own blind spots and biases.

Goals and Objectives Sought

Every intervention is based on a conception of the ends it is supposed to achieve. Given the temptation of dealing in generalities at this stage, the goals must be concretized. For example, a goal to enhance the nursing assistants' psychosocial practice would include the aim to provide knowledge and techniques to work with the residents' personal and interpersonal problems.

Characteristics of the Target Population

The characteristics of the target population, in this instance, the nursing assistants, must be described including their age, sex, ethnicity or race, education, level of skill, and turnover. This description may have been part of the problem statement. If not, it must be generated soon after and considered in relationship to the goals and possible interventions. Also, such elusive phenomena as the relations between the nursing assistants and other staff and residents should be considered.

Characteristics of the Helping Persons

The desired characteristics of helping persons--nursing educators, social-behavioral science consultants, researcher-evaluators--must be stated, especially if their contribution is to solve the defined problem. The greater the match between the helping persons and the demands of the problem, the greater the prospect of its solution.

Intervention Opportunities Are Identified

The persons engaged in initiating a change effort will almost always have a particular intervention in mind as they begin their planning. Moreover, they may have made a comparative analysis of various interventions very early in the process and have decided on a particular one.

Whatever may have occurred in the early considerations, it is highly important that several potential interventions be identified and these be weighed for their technical advantages and disadvantages, their cost, and their demand for personnel and facilities.

Problem May Be Redefined

The statement of a problem may remain intact throughout the planning--from the early consideration-speculation to the implementation of an intervention. However, it is not uncommon for the initial problem statement to be limited and perhaps parochial, particularly as the statement is reviewed and interfaced with potential remedies.

The essence of the problem statement must provide direction for the choice of an intervention and its specific design including the goals, objectives, and methods.

Construction of the Model

Using theory, research findings, experience, and logic, the intervention must zero in on the key dynamics of the problem to bring about the desired results. The overall strategy and immediate tactics and techniques must be set in place, and the necessary personnel, adjuncts, and props for the intervention must be specified. Scheduling the intervention effectiveness, especially in relationship to the characteristics of the subjects, is important, as is the development of the intervention techniques and plans to handle crises. Termination procedures and followup plans for the target population must also be indicated in advance. The plan to evaluate the intervention effectiveness and/or process must be built into the overall design of the project and must be structured to limit bias and unwanted influences on the process and outcome.

Implementation of the Model

Once constructed, the intervention must be carried out. This requires convincing the nursing home's major decision makers and the nursing assistants, if they have not been convinced already, of the intervention's usefulness. Involving these persons at an early point in the planning (if they were not the instigators of the idea) and presenting the major thrust of the plan candidly should ease the acceptance of a project.

Even with careful planning and involvement of all pertinent persons, unanticipated problems and resistances may emerge. These must be dealt with sensitively and thoroughly for the implementation to proceed. People's feelings and more objective matters must be worked out.

Monitoring the Model

The intervention must be monitored to be sure it is delivered as planned. Circumstances other than those envisioned during the planning may arise in the conduct of the intervention. Monitoring helps deliver the vision encompassed in the intervention and assist when trouble arises.

Evaluating the Model

Interventions require evaluation if they are to be improved. The particular evaluation design including its scope and direction must be tailored to the problem being addressed, the type of intervention being attempted, and the goals being sought.

TWO FORMS OF INSERVICE TRAINING TO ENHANCE THE PSYCHOSOCIAL COMPETENCE OF NURSING ASSISTANTS

Nursing assistants must have basic nursing knowledge and skill, understand their role and work relationships with other staff members, and have particular knowledge and skill pertaining to the residents' psychosocial needs (Almquist and Bates, 1980; Institute of Medicine, 1986; and the Omnibus Budget Reconciliation Act of 1987).

The nursing home typically provides some training to familiarize the nursing assistant with basic nursing care procedures and to orient them to their duties and responsibilities; however, it is unlikely to provide substantial training on the psychosocial aspects of resident care.

As indicated earlier, two models of inservice training will be presented: human relations and behavioral. Both training models have the same goals, curriculum materials, and organizational format. Both approaches--human relations and behavioral--seek the same goal in their training: to improve the psychosocial competence of nursing assistants to care for residents. The general areas of competence include the ability to identify the residents' manner of thinking (including thought disorder), feelings, and relationships (with peers, family, and nursing assistants); and skills to help the residents with their thinking, feelings, and relationships.

Detail on these items includes the nursing assistants' skill in identifying and dealing with the residents':

Feelings, affective states, and disorders, including excessive anxiety, fear, dependency, boredom, anger, jealousy, loneliness, sadness, and depression.

Thought processes, including lack of attention and concentration, confusion and loss of memory, self-doubt and obsessions, suspiciousness, wildly false accusations, delusions, and hallucinations.

Interpersonal relations with each other, such as friendliness, argument, intimidation, physical threat, constant hassles, gossip, and breaking up friendships.

Interpersonal relations with nursing assistants, such as congeniality and friendliness, complaints about nursing assistants' services and about the general program, challenges to nursing assistants' authority, and excessive demands on nursing assistants.

Interpersonal relations with family, including quarrels and strained relationships, abandonment, and the family's pressing to acquire resident's possessions.

Conditions of special care, for example, incontinence and total care.

The two training models would use the same case materials as a part of the curriculum. These are drawn from Weber and McCall (1987). Both models would have: a nurse, highly knowledgeable about resident care and skilled in either human relations or behavioral psychology, as the instructor; a small number of nursing assistants (ten to twelve) enrolled to facilitate discussion; fifteen one-and-a-half-hour classes, spread over fifteen weeks; a brief introductory lecture at the beginning of every class on the topic to be considered; and a summary at the close of the class. The instructors of both models should write lesson plans to concretize the teaching procedures.

The topics of the classes follow.

Session 1, 2, and 3: Styles of residents' mental functioning (Weber and McCall, pp. 57-88).

The specific topics and cases:

Confusion and disorientation: Mr. Palmer and his brother. Mr. Shaw and his memory.

Suspicion and accusations: Mr. Mills and Coke. Mrs. Wilbur and Room 265.

Delusions and hallucinations: Mrs. Gatewood and chronicity. Mrs. Lawler and electric waves.

Avoidance and denial: Cora Armstrong's children and relatives. Mr. Redmond's correctional surgery.

Displacement: Gertrude's messiness. Mrs. Jones' complaints.

Session 4 and 5: Kinds of residents' distressed feelings. (Weber and McCall, pp. 25-56).

The specific topics and cases are:

Loneliness: Mrs. Galt's family has rejected him. Mary Cook's loneliness causes a perceptual distortion.

Anxiety and fear: Mrs. Barnes and traffic noises. Mrs. Curtis' anxiety continues on and off. Mr. Grant: spending money and fear. Dora and the lift machine.

Anger and hostility: Mr. Southwell's explosive anger. Miss Johnson's underlying anger and jealousy.

Unfounded bodily complaints: Mrs. Beam and women's troubles. Mr. Stout's need for recognition.

(Sadness, depression, and suicide will be considered in Session 14).

Sessions 6-11: Kinds of resident relationships, particularly those generating stress between the residents and staff, and between residents and their family. (Weber and McCall, pp. 89-106). Details on the class sessions 6-11 follow:

Sessions 6 and 7: Relationships and stress among the residents. The specific topics and cases are:

Argument: Mrs. Roark and Mrs. Flowers and their room's temperature. Grandma Harper and the postcard.

Intimidation by attitude: Mr. Ross and Mrs. Cooley and intimidation.

Physical threat: Mr. Reynolds and his cane. Mr. Miller and shuffleboard.

Lack of interest: Mr. Steward and his roommate. Nellie is despondent.

Constant hassle: Mr. Lyon and argument. Mrs. Grey and Mrs. Hobbs and earrings.

Sessions 8 and 9: Relationships and stress between residents and nursing assistants. (Weber and McCall, pp. 127-144)

The specific topics and cases are:

Complaints about service and care: Mr. Johnson at a Residents' Council Meeting. Lorrie Parsons and lack of cooperation.

Challenging the Staff: Mr. Sullivan and cigarettes. Josephine, Zelda and Elaine--and crowding.

Blunders and abuse: Mrs. Starr and awareness. Mr. Merton and the staff pledge.

Complaints about the program: Mrs. Yale, the Bingo Group, and a prospective literary group. Mr. Beker and the volunteer party. Mrs. Holt and call lights. Virginia Pardes and complaining.

Sessions 10 and 11: Relations and stress among residents and family. (Weber and McCall, pp. 145-165).

The specific topics and cases are:

Neglect: Mr. James Hilton and mechanical relationships. Mrs. Crosby and staying.

Abandonment: Marjorie Calvert and Georgette Wilson, on being useful.   William Adams has been deserted.

Possessions: Mrs. Margarite Aster and jewelry.   Mr. Chern is down.

Demands: Mrs. Vernon and visits.   Mr. and Mrs. Ewing and snacks.

Uncertainty: Mr. Webb and his son.   Mr. Walter and family complications.

Sessions 12-14:   Special care situations (Weber & McCall, pp. 167-220; for sadness, depression, and suicide, pp. 51-56).

The specific topics and cases are:

Belongings: Mrs. Timbers and missing items.   Mr. Huron's blue shirt.

Resident noncompliance: Mr. Helms and medicine.   Mrs. Landman and her hearing aid.

Sexual interest: Grover and Bessy: petting.   Clint and Anabel and their attachment.

Selfish and self-indulgent residents: Mrs. Parker and her pattern.   Mrs. Averill and her winnings.

Mentally ill residents: Penelope Diction and Carrie.   Mr. Pace and real estate.

Lack of Cleanliness: Mrs. Hodges and odor.   Mrs. Hanks and bathing.

Incontinence: Mrs. Harris and help.   Miss Rooney and Mrs. Connell discuss heavy care.

Death and dying: Mr. Darwin has gone downhill.   Mr. Norris' anger.

Sadness, depression and suicide: Mr. Cressey's stubborn depression.   Mrs. Coleman's depression and delusions.   Blanche Becker's suicide.

Session 15:   Many things to feel good about.   Emphasis on nursing assistants' sensitivity and skill.   (Weber and McCall, pp. 209-224).

The specific topics and cases are:

The Importance of the work: Picking up where no one else can.   Mrs. Hooper doesn't recognize me.   Pride in a job well done.   Mrs. Hart and new shoes.   Friends.

SPECIFICS ON HUMAN RELATIONS TRAINING

Educational Theories Underlying the Human Relations Model

Of particular theoretical relevance to the human relations model is the social psychology of Kurt Lewin (1942) and the ideas of Elton Mayo (1945) and Mary Follett (1940). Lewin encouraged the use of group discussion to change attitudes and behavior. Miles (1959) used Lewin's approach to train various kinds of groups, especially teachers. He urged a particular learning process, including the group members' identifying common problems, selecting new or modified approaches, practicing the new modified approaches, implementing these approaches, and refining their use in practice. Mayo and Follett reasoned that the case method of teaching is an insightful way of communicating problem-solving skills. Further, they suggested that the case method encourages learners to work inductively from the case material to a more general understanding, and from that understanding to remediation, if such is indicated.

Procedural Detail of the Human Relations Model

The style of the human relations instructor should be friendly, facilitative, and encouraging to engage the nursing assistants in considering the care challenges in the case and bringing their experience to bear on it. Also, the instructor's style must encourage the nursing assistants to solve case problems as well as to identify them and their dynamics, and to generalize from the specifics of cases to general principles.

After giving a substantive introductory lecture, the instructor will have the nursing assistants choose the cases they want to discuss as a means of involving them in the process and have the nursing assistants summarize the class session before closing.

SPECIFICS ON BEHAVIORAL TRAINING

Psychological Theories Underlying the Behavioral Model

The ideas underlying the behavioral model stem mainly from Skinner's (1968) contentions that the crucial events from which we predict and control behavior are environmental stimuli, and that behavior is strengthened or weakened by the immediate consequences that follow--reinforcement and extinction. Reinforcement means the strengthening of various behavioral responses through rewards. Extinction pertains to wiping out a particular behavior or response by punishment. In addition to Skinner's contribution to behavioral training is Bandura's (1977) conception of social learning--that a person's learning is determined by a reciprocal interaction between person and environment. Further, Bandura suggested that the vast majority of behavior is acquired through observing and copying others, that is, modeling behavior after others. Another contribution was Wolpe's (1958) concept of counterconditioning, especially its emphasis on substituting a skillful for an unskillful response (in this instance, a skillful nursing assistant response to a resident's problem in contrast to an unskilled one).

Procedural Detail of the Behavioral Model

The behavioral model, like the human relations model, aims to improve the nursing assistants' psychosocial knowledge and skills for resident care.

The style of the behavioral instructor should be friendly and instructive to teach the knowledge and skills of psychosocial care. Following his introductory lecture, the instructor will analyze the cases of his choosing to demonstrate and model case analysis and planning for the nursing assistants. When the instructor judges an appropriate amount of instruction has been given, she will ask the nursing assistants questions about the case analysis and planning and then have them proceed with such on the cases. The instructor will use verbal support and praise to reinforce their positive responses, and verbal discouragement to rule out their inadequate and incorrect ones. Also, the instructor will provide a summary at the close of each class on the major points covered.

Evaluation

Evaluation of training is encouraged. The character of the evaluation, whether it seeks to describe the program and its apparent effects or whether it seeks to test a program more rigorously for its effectiveness, is determined by the design of the program and the method of the evaluation. Though the rigor of the training and its evaluation influence the credibility of the evaluation's findings, qualitative descriptive reports as well as statistical analyses conducted on quasi-experimental programs can contribute to understanding training programs and their results. Projects of exceptional rigor might contribute to the technology of training. That prospect is enhanced if the evaluations compare different types of training and use objective research procedures.

TWO FORMS OF ORGANIZATIONAL DEVELOPMENT TO ENHANCE THE PSYCHOSOCIAL COMPETENCE OF NURSING ASSISTANTS

Organizations, including nursing homes, have their various components: leadership; hierarchical arrangement of positions; division of work; communication; supervision and coordination; and dos and don'ts backed up by a set of values, rewards, and punishments. It is in this network that the work of the nursing assistant takes place.

Ideally the various aspects of the nursing home organization fit the nursing assistant's modes of orientation, that is, their information and skills, emotional attachments, typical types of action, and values. Usually the fit between the organization and the individual is only approximate. However, there are organizational policies and procedures to inform the nursing assistant and influence her action in regard to assessing and responding to the needs of the residents. Yet such policies and procedures are typically underdeveloped (Institute of Medicine, 1986).

Organizational development seeks to improve organizations through planned, systematic efforts focused on their culture and its various processes (French and Bell, 1984). Its objectives are to make the organization more effective, more viable, and better able to achieve the goals of the organization and the goals of individuals in the organization. Its procedures include team building, consultation, structural reorganization, strategic management activities, planning and goal setting, coaching and counseling, and education and training.

Two forms of organizational development are considered: a staff-directed model and a consultant-conducted model. Both organizational development model share a theory, goals, and some procedures.

Kurt Lewin's (1942) conceptions of the "force field" and "quasi-stationary equilibrium" underlie the several strategies of change that guide the two organizational development plans. Force field refers to the driving and restraining forces in a situation that effect some type of organizational change. Quasi-stationary equilibrium reflects the dynamic as well as the static condition of a situation. Thus while a situation typically has considerable stability, it is not motionless or impermeable to influence.

The goals of both models are to improve the policies and procedures governing the nursing assistants' psychosocial practice. The policies and procedures must help the nursing assistants identify the residents' manner of functioning, and engage appropriate skills to work with it; for example, the residents' manner of thinking (including thought disorder), feelings and affective disorders, and manner of relating to peers, family, and nursing assistants. Another goal of the development efforts is to involve the nursing assistants in the policy process of the nursing home, especially the policies on nursing care.

These goals require that records and documents of the nursing homes be studied, and that knowledgeable persons be interviewed. Not only should the pertinent formal written policies and procedures be identified, but the unwritten ones as well. Past and current policies and procedures must be analyzed for their treatment of nursing assistants' responsibilities to deal with the residents' feelings, thoughts, relationships, and disorders in these areas.

After the above analysis is completed, the staff director or the consultant (depending on which model is being employed), with others involved, must formulate policies and procedures to enhance the nursing assistants' psychosocial practice, including their skills in dealing with various aspects of the residents' functioning that were detailed in the previous section on inservice training models. Those aspects of functioning included feelings, thought processes, interpersonal relations, and the conditions of special care.

Next, the project director (staff director or consultant) and involved staff must develop their plans to implement the new policies and procedures. Get the nursing home administrator's approval to proceed. The plans to implement must consider the possible resistance to effect change and the limitations of the nursing home resources.

The actual implementation should move quickly and decisively. Though some changes may have occurred in the process of conducting the project, announcements and manuals containing the new and revised policies and procedures governing the nursing assistants must be issued.

Specifics on the Staff-Directed Model

The staff-directed model draws on empirical-rational, normative reeducative, and power-coercive concepts for change (Chin and Benne, 1985). The empirical-rational concept suggests that the administration of the nursing home consider its staff to be rational and willing to follow their rational self-interest. The normative reeducative strategy indicates the staff are able to change as they are exposed to education that alters their normative orientations to old patterns and develops commitments to new ones, including changes in attitudes, values, skills, and relationships to others. The power-coercive strategy though typically cast in soft language compels by pressure or threat of force to effect organizational development.

Having a mandate from the administrator, the staff member designated to head the organization's development may proceed with authority. Her actions to assemble people, make assignments, set deadlines, generate policies and procedures, and initiate action should be decisive. This does not mean she has carte blanche, as the administrator will require consultation and clearance of particular actions; however, within that parameter, she has the authority to move. Further, being in the organization's line of authority, the designated staff member has access to such resources as the production and distribution of documents, the nursing home's communication system, and its richness of information. In addition, being in the organization makes her cognizant of its values, norms, and decision-making procedures, all of which are highly relevant to getting something done. Finally, the designated staff member, with the approval of the administrator and in some instances the concurrence of the nursing home's appropriate department heads, may make personnel changes and reformulate parts of the organization to bring about a set of policies and procedures.

Specifics on the Consultant-Conducted Model

The consultant-conducted model is based on a mix of conceptions; a normative reeducative strategy is the major one. The empirical-rational perspective is another, especially its team building, staff development, and effort to influence group processes. The authority concept used explicitly in the staff-directed model may be used occasionally by this model, if agreed to by the administrator--for example, if the planned activities were not working out as anticipated and other techniques of the consultant were unsuccessful.

Even though the consultant may have a modicum of authority that flows from her agreement or contract with the nursing home, her main authority stems from her expertise (knowledge and skill about the psychosocial care of the elderly and policy development) and her leadership. She will use techniques such as: involving the staff in generating and analyzing data and considering their implications for change; planning through task forces; developing a team spirit by encouraging the staff to participate in the organizational effort; and offering staff training. Also, she will confer, advise, share information, suggest, and pursuade. Further, the consultant must liaison actively with the administrator to be sure they agree on the proceedings of the organization's development.

The nursing home staff's view of an outsider may vary. The staff may distrust an outsider. On the other hand, they may trust the consultant because she is not an integral part of the nursing home hierarchy. Much depends on the disposition of the staff and the personality of the consultant.

Finally, whether an organizational development effort is lead by a consultant or an in-house staff member, the effort is likely to encounter significant resistance. Yet the consultant, not having institutional authority and having a time-limited contract, is less able to deal with the resistance than a staff member, who has access to power if not possessing it herself.

Evaluation

Qualitative methods are particularly appropriate to study an organization as complex as a nursing home. Yet, certain aspects of this study might be quantified--for example, the number of new policies that were written--and these might be related to various features of the development effort. With exceptional research planning, comparative evaluations of different ways of developing a nursing home might be carried out. The circumstances would require having two comparable nursing homes, each using a different model and employing the same research methods.

A FORM OF ADVOCACY AND A FORM OF BARGAINING

The procedures of advocacy and bargaining are typically interrelated, though each can be defined as a discrete procedure or technique.

Advocacy is the act of stating one's own case or that of another, citing an issue, pleading a cause, and asking for correction based on some concept of justice, for example, equity (Weber and McCall, 1978). It is used by (among other professionals) lawyers, who investigate and organize the facts of a case and represent their clients in court and other settings, and by social workers, who speak and lobby on behalf of their clients.

When advocacy fails to be effective in such matters as improving wages and working conditions, bargaining may join the process. A general concept of bargaining (Bacharach and Lawler, 1981) includes: two bargainers who are virtually stuck in their relationship; an issue confronting them that is conceptualized as the distribution of some quantitative resource; and a negotiation that has the potential for several different settlements.

Given the vested interests of nursing assistants and the owners and managers of nursing homes, the likelihood of structuring models of advocacy and bargaining for testing is exceptionally small, if possible at all. Yet studies might be conducted on naturally occurring advocacy or bargaining, provided the necessary permissions are obtained from the parties involved. Such advocacy and bargaining by nursing assistants are likely to be direct, unsophisticated, and reasonable. Here such advocacy is entitled a "straightforward style of advocacy"; and a comparable style of bargaining is called a "rational-equity model of bargaining."

Advocacy and bargaining are likely to be conducted for higher wages, improved working conditions, greater involvement in the nursing home's decision making about the residents' care, and perhaps inservice training. These items are usually viewed as fair in terms of community standards for workers, and necessary to improve the residents' care.

A Straightforward Style of Advocacy

The projected advocacy anticipates: a consensus among the nursing assistants, or a substantial number of them, on the definition of their problems; data having been collected on them, or definite plans having been made to do so; a commitment among the nursing assistants to proceed with their case; the emergence of a leader among the nursing assistants; and a thoughtful response from the administration. The style of the advocacy will be informal, serious, direct, matter of fact, and persistent.

Advocacy with Organizational Legitimacy

It is projected that such advocacy takes place in a nursing home that not only allows advocacy by nursing assistants but also provides such mechanisms as a committee or panel and administrative lines to consider the nursing assistants' interests.

As suggested earlier, the nursing assistants must meet together prior to gathering facts, to decide how they want to state their problem, what facts they need to gather and possible ways to proceed. Once the facts are gathered and the initial tactics decided on, the nursing assistants should be ready to meet with the appropriate facility official to present their concern and explore the facility's position.

Their case is likely to be "heard out" if the style is serious, thorough, and explicit. Though intrusive because of its very nature, advocacy need not be belligerent. Advocacy is a process. A single presentation is unlikely to produce the desired results. Most cases require followup efforts, perhaps with additional information and the involvement of other people, giving the administration time to consider the request but pursuing the administration doggedly and respectfully.

Though administrators and boards of nursing homes prefer smooth-running organizations--ones without compelling dissatisfaction or strife--they allow, and in some limited instances welcome, the advocacy of their staff. An office or committee may be set up to accommodate the staff's concerns. The residents will be best served if the staff's concerns about their jobs are given serious consideration.

If the nursing assistants have a problem, they do not have to speculate about how to find their way into the hierarchy; however, the actual route to the "desk of resolution," and whom to involve (and when) to gain the most favorable consideration are likely to be more complicated than indicated on the nursing home's organizational chart. The help of coalitions, informal contacts with major decision makers, strategic timing of the advocacy, and the substantive quality of the appeal are likely to influence the outcome of the effort.

Advocacy Without Facility Legitimacy

If a nursing home does not recognize the nursing assistants' right to advocate in their own behalf, or does so grudgingly, the nursing assistants' right to make a request or express a grievance is considerably limited. The seriousness of their problem may propel them to review their own strengths; for example, their knowledge of the home's organization, their skill in developing and organizing information, and their ability to present and argue an issue of concern. The nursing assistants are advised to seek help from outside sources, especially from the nurses.

BARGAINING

Bargaining typically involves a union negotiator representing the nursing assistants and a member of the nursing home administration, or a negotiator representing the administration. The two parties will have divergent interests, for example, on wages, fringe benefits, and working conditions. Yet the parties are usually able to communicate and often to compromise. Provisional offers may be made in the course of the bargaining; however, their terms do not fix any part of the final agreement until they are accepted by both sides.

Bargaining is concerned with practical matters such as wages, numbers of residents to be cared for, and so on. Yet theories have been constructed to explain bargaining, or certain aspects of it. For example, bargaining by an aggrieved party seeks equity or strives to achieve a particular level of aspiration (Adams, 1965).

Nash (1950) set forth a number of assumptions about the elements of the relationship between the bargainers:

Actors are rational and expect others to be rational.

Actors attempt to maximize their own gain or utility.

Actors have complete information on the utility of alternative settlements to themselves and their opponent.

Neither party will settle for an agreement that is not optimal-- preferable in comparison to all possible outcomes.

"Good faith" bargaining--once a bargainer makes an offer it cannot be retracted, and an agreement, once reached, is enforceable.

If final demands or offers are incompatible and rejected, the bargaining is not only terminated but destroyed, except if the termination is by mutual consent, instead of open hostility, in which case the likelihood of reconstituting the bargaining is enhanced.

A Rational-Equity Model of Bargaining

Theoretical Basis

The proposed model of bargaining is based on equity theory (Adams and Freedman, 1976). At the center of the theory lies the rule that judgments about justice must reflect the relative ratio of one's contributions to one's receipts. Further, the rule indicates that justice is achieved when this ratio appears equal for all individuals involved in a given distribution or exchange.

Other tenents of equity theory are: people try to maximize their receipts, that is, they try to get as much as possible; and perceptions of inequity cause distress and inhibit efforts to achieve equity (Walster, Walster, and Berschied, 1978).

Also, the current model is based on the distributive theory of justice, which holds that all social interactions involve the exchange of rewards and punishments among individuals or groups. On this point, bargaining has rules and procedures for the fair allocation of rewards and punishments.

Procedures of the Model

This theoretical background implies that by collecting objective data on the issue (wages, working conditions, and so on) and comparing these data with similar data on other workers doing comparable work, a case for inequity can be made. This case for inequity should also include illustrative materials to dramatize the data and give them reality. Further, the distributive perspective (using rules and procedures for fair distribution) suggests that bargaining should proceed under the conditions of the Labor Management Relations Act, 1947, as amended by subsequent public laws, which include the right of employees to organize and bargain collectively.

Rationality and good faith are basic to bargaining. Rationality includes knowing the opposition. For the nursing assistants this requires that they have knowledge of the administration's stance on the issues and the settlements it might entertain, and the possible consequences of these settlements. The nursing assistants' preparation, presentation, and bargaining should be matter of fact, psychologically aware, and persistent. Rationality also includes presenting a data-based, objective case that they believe is superior to other alternatives.

Good faith points two ways: one to bargaining, that it will produce the desired results; and another to the administration, that it will be persuaded by the reasonableness of the demand.

Other elements are also a part of bargaining. The administration may attribute a lower value than the nursing assistants do to their work; not consider a pay raise as economically feasible as the nursing assistants do; and emotions and personality eccentricities may be a factor.

EVALUATION

Detailed descriptive evaluation of advocacy and bargaining should identify and describe the various aspects of these procedures and trace some of their relationships. Given the complex, illusive, and qualitative nature of advocacy and bargaining, detailed description will help pin down their elements, and reflect their contribution to the outcomes. Comparative studies in which a particular type of advocacy or bargaining would be tested for their effectiveness in two different circumstances might be attempted.

SUMMARY

This chapter presented six models to improve the psychosocial practice of nursing assistants--human relations and behavioral models in training, staff-directed and consultant-conducted organizational development models, and advocacy and bargaining models. In addition, the various factors to consider in planning a model were discussed.

VII
Additional Considerations

The circle has been rounded. The first four chapters presented the annotations of the literature on the nursing assistants' job, their work environment, organizational development, training, and advocacy and bargaining. The choice of the literature was influenced by the intent to construct model interventions to improve the psychosocial practice of nursing assistants. The four chapters containing the annotations were followed by a chapter that presented a psychosocial model of practice. Next, Chapter 6 suggested program models to improve the psychosocial practice of nursing assistants including inservice training, organizational development, and advocacy and bargaining.

Though the circle has been rounded it may not have been sufficiently inclusive. In addition to the items already noted, the nursing assistant occupation requires development.

That undertaking requires initiative from the nursing assistants and others in the nursing home and outside of it including foundations, unions, and universities. The necessary activities, in addition to the technical developments that have been discussed, are political. Regulations must be revised to improve the standards of training and practice. Influence must be exercised to improve salaries, benefits, and the conditions of work.

The behavior of nursing assistants has not been political, perhaps to the contrary. They do not have a record of running for elected office, doing campaign work, making financial contributions, or articulating their voting. The lack of a political tradition, and of self-confidence and psychic security to enter the political arena, contribute to this nonparticipation.

Politicians and others have expressed concern about the plight of nursing assistants; however, only as part of a larger matter: the long-term care of the elderly. The interests of nursing assistants are further skewed by the political agendas of the nursing home owners, operators, and professionals that are unlikely to give priority to the needs and contributions of nursing assistants.

Prerequisite actions may be necessary before the nursing assistants can become politically active. They must begin to solidify their occupation by setting standards of practice, constructing a code of ethics, developing a standard curriculum of training, certifying their members for competency, building an occupational association to provide leadership, and by unionizing their members for collective bargaining and associated activities.

Yet political activity must not await the achievement of all the foregoing actions. Minimally, the nursing assistants must get sufficiently well organized to proceed with confidence, which means they also must get equipped with a program of occupational and political relevance, and personal skills to present it.

The training models--human relations and behavioral--and the organizational development models--staff-directed and consultant-conducted--should contribute to developing standards of practice and training curriculum, and contribute indirectly to solidifying the occupation, and perhaps identifying issues to be considered in writing a code of ethics.

The advocacy and bargaining models embody ideas that should be directly useful in solidifying the occupation, developing standards of practice, and unionizing the members. Also, the models contain ideas that may be used to approach a wide variety of problems faced by nursing assistants.

Along with the question of how to proceed is the matter of who shall lead. The demanding work life of the nursing assistants and their unfamiliarity with the tasks and techniques of building an occupation may limit the probability of an indigenously lead movement. However, that prospect should not be ruled out, especially if the nursing assistants were to receive the active, yet carefully gauged guidance of an outside group such as a foundation, a union, or an action-advocacy agency.

Another unmentioned dimension to the undeveloped character of the nursing assistants practice that should be considered is the moral dimension. Benne (1985) wrote that a manager's responsibilities have a moral quality. That is, the responsibilities have serious effects on the worker's quality of life. Administrators (and the boards and owners) of nursing homes have a moral obligation to train, upgrade, and compensate the nursing assistants for the services they provide. This obligation cannot be avoided, denied, or finessed. Excuses such as "not enough time," "not enough money," "not enough expertise," and "we're doing fine the way we are" are not only inadequate, they are inappropriate.

Given the residents' substantial need for psychosocial attention and the nursing assistants' immediacy to the residents' daily life, nursing assistants should be trained and sanctioned to provide psychosocial care, and given appropriate support. To do little or nothing about this need and opportunity is not only to let an opportunity to do good slide; it is licentious. It is knowingly to let the residents' psychosocial needs go unattended, excepting as they are indirectly and inadequately met by the nursing home's general program.

SUMMARY

Political and moral actions were considered as necessary to generate improved nursing assistant psychosocial practice. Political action is necessary by several groups including the nursing assistants, although they have not had such a tradition. The initiative to improve the nursing assistants' psychosocial care, and the lack of such, have a moral quality. That is, to act is moral, to fail to act is immoral. Much of this lies with the administrator, boards, and owners of nursing homes.

References

INTRODUCTION

Institute of Medicine (1986). <u>Improving the quality of nursing homes</u>. Washington, D.C.: National Academy Press.
National Citizens' Coalition for Nursing Home Reform (NCCNHR). (1988). <u>Final report, Nurses aide training symposium</u>. Washington, D.C.: NCCNHR.

CHAPTER 1

<u>Culmulative index to nursing and allied health literature</u>. (volumes 1980-1988). Glendale, Calif.: Glendale Adventist Medical Center.
Dissertation Abstracts International (volumes 1971-1986). <u>A. Humanities and social sciences; B. Physical sciences and engineering</u>. Ann Arbor, Mich.: Dissertation Publishing, University Microfilms International.
Institute of Medicine (1986). <u>Improving the quality of nursing homes</u>. Washington, D.C.: National Academy Press.
National Citizens' Coalition for Nursing Home Reform (NCCNHR). (1988). <u>Final report, Nurse aide training symposium</u>. Washington, D.C.: NCCNHR.
National Council on the Aging (volumes 1980-1989). <u>Current literature on aging</u>. Washington, D.C.: National Council on the Aging.

CHAPTER 5

Almquist, E., and Bates, D. (1980). "Training program for nursing assistants and LPNs in nursing homes." <u>Journal of Gerontological Nursing</u>, 6(10):622-627.

Biddle, B. J., and Thomas, E. J. (1966). Role theory: Concepts and research. New York: John Wiley and Sons.

Blau, D., and Freed, A. D. (editors) (1979). Mental health in the nursing home: An educational program for staff. Brookline, Mass.: Boston Society for Gerontologic Psychiatry Incorporated.

Brannon, D., et al. (1988). "A job diagnostic survey of nursing home caregivers: Implications for job redesign." The Gerontologist, 28(2):246-252.

Bye, M. G., and Iannone, J. (1987). "Excellent care-givers of the elderly: What satisfies them about their work." Nursing Homes, 36(4):36-39.

Dawes, P. L. (1981). "The nurses' aide and the team approach in the nursing home." Journal of Geriatric Psychiatry, 14(2):265-276.

Fisk, V. R. (1984). "When nurses aides care." Journal of Gerontological Nursing, 10(3):121-127.

Gale, C. B. (1973). "Walking in the aide's shoes." American Journal of Nursing, 73(4):628-631.

Handschu, S. S. (1973). "Profile of the nurse's aide: Expanding her role as psycho-social companion to the nursing home resident." The Gerontologist, 31(17):315-317.

Institute of Medicine (1986). Improving the quality of nursing homes. Washington, D.C.: National Academy Press.

Klus, G. W., and Thoreson, E. H. (1980). "The nurse aide: A life of uncertainty." Nursing Homes, 29(2):2-8.

LeSar, K. W. (1987). "Who provides for the nursing assistant?". Provider, 13(4):20-22.

Likert, R. (1967). The human organization. New York: McGraw-Hill.

Mueller, D. J., and Atlas, L. (1972). "Resocialization of regressed elderly residents: A behavioral management approach." Journal of Gerontology, 27(3):390-392.

National Citizens' Coalition for Nursing Home Reform (NCCNHR). (1988). Nurses aide training symposium: Final report. Washington, D.C.: NCCNHR.

Rinke, C. L., Williams, J. J., Lloyd, K. E., and Smith-Scott, W. (1978). "The effects of prompting and reinforcement on self-bathing by elderly residents of a nursing home." Behavioral Therapy, 9(5):873-881.

Sand, P., and Berni, R. (1974). "An incentive contract for nursing home aides." American Journal of Nursing, 74(3):475-477.

Schnelle, J. F., and Traughber, B. (1983). "A behavioral assessment system applicable to geriatric nursing facility residents." Behavioral Assessment, 5(3):231-243.

Wagnild, G., and Manning, R. W. (1986). "Screening and selecting applicants for nurse's aide." The Journal of Long-Term Care Administration, 14(2):2-4.

Weber, G. H., and McCall, G. J. (1987). The nursing assistant's casebook of elder care. Dover, Mass.: Auburn House.

CHAPTER 6

Adams, J. S., and Freedman, S. (1976). "Equity theory revisited: Comments and annotated bibliography." In Berkowitz, L. (editor), Advances in experimental social psychology, vol. 2. New York: Academic Press.

Adams, J. S. (1965). "Inequity in social exchange." In Berkowitz, L. (editor), Advances in experimental social psychology, vol 2. New York: Academic Press.

Almquist, E., and Bates, D. (1980). "Training program for nursing assistants and LPNs in nursing homes." Journal of Gerontological Nursing, 6(10):622-627.

Bacharach, S. B., and Lawler, E. J. (1981). Bargaining: Power, tactics, and outcomes. San Francisco: Jossey-Bass.

Bandura, A. (1977). Social learning theory. Englewood Cliffs, N.J.: Prentice-Hall.

Chin, R., and Benne, K. D. (1985). "General strategies for effecting changes in human systems." In Bennis, W. G., Benne, K. D., and Chin, R. (editors), The planning of change. 312 Pp. Fourth edition. New York: Holt, Rinehart & Winston.

Follett, M. P. (1940). Dynamic administration: The collected papers of Mary Parker Follett, edited by Metcalf, H. C., and Urwick, L. New York: Harper & Row.

Institute of Medicine. (1986). Improving the quality of care in nursing homes. Washington, D.C.: National Academy Press.

Knowles, M. (1984). Third edition. The adult learner: A neglected species. Houston: Gulf.

Lewin, K. (1942). "Field theory and learning: The psychology of learning." Forty-first Yearbook of the National Society for the Study of Education, Part II. Chicago: University of Chicago Press.

Mayo, E. (1945). The social problems of an industrial civilization. Cambridge: Harvard University Press.

Miles, M. B. (1959). Learning to work in groups. New York: Teachers College Press.

Myrdal, G. (1944). An American dilemma: The negro problem and modern democracy. New York: Harper and Brothers.

Nash, J. F., Jr. (1950). "The bargaining problem." Econometrica, 18(2):155-162.

Omnibus Budget Reconciliation Act of 1987.

Skinner, B. F. (1968). The technology of teaching. New York: Appleton.

Walster, E., Walster, G. W., and Berscheid, E. (1978). Equity: Theory and research. Boston, Mass.: Allyn and Bacon.

Weber, G. H., and McCall, G. J. (1987). The nursing assistant's casebook of elder care. Dover, Mass.: Auburn House.

Weber, G. H., and McCall, G. J. (editors) (1978). Social scientists as advocates: Views from the applied disciplines. Beverly Hills, Calif.: Sage.

Wolpe, J. (1958). Psychotherapy by reciprocal inhibition. Stanford, Calif.: Stanford University Press.

CHAPTER 7

Benne, K. D. (1985). "Moral dilemmas of managers." In Bennis, W. G., Benne, K. D., and Chin, R. (editors), The planning of change. Fourth edition, New York: Holt, Rinehart & Winston.

Author Index

Subject Index

About the Author

GEORGE H. WEBER is Professor in the National School of Social Service at The Catholic University of America. He is co-author of *Nursing Assistant's Casebook of Eldercare* (Auburn House, 1987) and *Social Science and Public Policy*. He has also written many articles on various aspects of human behavior.